A Manual of Clinical Hysteroscopy

A Manual of Clinical Hysteroscopy

Rafael F. Valle, MD

Professor, Department of Obstetrics and Gynecology
Northwestern University Medical School
Chicago, IL, USA

Foreword by

John J. Sciarra, MD, PhD

Thomas J. Watkins Professor and Chair
Department of Obstetrics and Gynecology
Northwestern University Medical School
Chicago, IL, USA

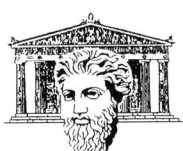

The Parthenon Publishing Group
International Publishers in Medicine, Science & Technology

NEW YORK   LONDON

Library of Congress Cataloging-in-Publication Data
Valle, Rafael F.
      A manual of clinical hysteroscopy / Rafael F. Valle.
          p. cm. -- (Gynecological endoscopy manual series)
      Includes bibliographical references and index.
      ISBN 1-85070-641-7
      1. Hysteroscopy--Handbooks, manuals, etc. I. Title. II. Series.
      [DNLM: 1. Hysteroscopy. 2. Uterine Diseases--diagnosis.
      3. Uterine Diseases--therapy.   WP 440 V181m 1997]
      RG304.5.H97V35 1997
      618.1'4--dc21
      DNLM/DLC
      for Library of Congress   97–118022
                                                                CIP
British Library Cataloguing in Publication Data
Valle, Rafael F.
      A manual of clinical hysteroscopy. - (Gynecological endoscopy
      manual series)
      1. Hysteroscopy - Handbooks, manuals, etc. 2. Uterus - Diseases -
      Diagnosis - Handbooks, manuals, etc.
      I. Title
      618.1'4'07545

      ISBN 1-85070-641-7

Published in the USA by
The Parthenon Publishing Group Inc.
One Blue Hill Plaza
PO Box 1564, Pearl River
New York 10965, USA

Published in the UK and Europe by
The Parthenon Publishing Group
    Limited
Casterton Hall, Carnforth
Lancs. LA6 2LA, UK

Copyright ©1998
Parthenon Publishing Group

Printed and bound in Spain by
T.G. Hostench, S.A.

Contents

Dedication

To my teachers, my family and my patients,
who have kept me focused towards achieving my
intended objective

Foreword

Hysteroscopy is a dynamic and essential part of contemporary gynecological practice. *A Manual of Clinical Hysteroscopy* by Dr Rafael Valle is a wonderful concise and comprehensive practical text which covers both diagnostic and operative hysteroscopy.

The possibility of visualizing the interior of the uterus has interested physicians for the past 100 years. Hysteroscopy, however, did not become a standard reproducible clinical procedure until the advent of modern instrumentation. This manual is a fully illustrated and well-written presentation of the instruments and techniques that have evolved over the past two decades. The content is designed to serve as both a resource for the physician who is currently using hysteroscopy and also as an introductory text for those who are in the process of developing their skills with the technique.

In many ways, this book represents the cumulative experience and career of its author, Dr Valle, who is recognized to be one of the senior international authorities and leaders in the field of hysteroscopy and hysteroscopic surgery. Through his current position as a professor of obstetrics and gynecology at Northwestern University Medical School in Chicago, he has through the years personally taught the skills and techniques of diagnostic hysteroscopy and operative hysteroscopy to a large number of residents and practitioners. With this manual, we now have available to us the didactic material compiled over his many years of teaching hysteroscopy. The readers of this book, whether they be young physicians, accomplished practitioners or enthusiasts, will all benefit from the practical and useful guidelines developed by this one man who has had over 25 years of clinical experience in this field.

One of the best features of this book is its readability. A further plus is the continuity of presentation, as virtually all of the material has been prepared by the same author, with the exception of the four chapters on the various imaging modalities and pathology written by experts in those fields.

All invasive procedures must be accompanied by appropriate indications. Another strength of this text is its comprehensive presentation of the indications and contraindications for hysteroscopy. Although complications from the procedure are rare, it remains important that the practitioner be aware of the possible complications. Indeed, this book contains an excellent chapter on the subject.

Following a chapter devoted to office hysteroscopy, the reader is led into the exciting field of surgical hysteroscopic therapy. In these chapters, the author presents a clear and conservative portrayal of the value of operative hysteroscopic procedures, drawing from the available evidence as well as on his own extensive and practical experience.

Finally, this manual includes some excellent photographs of typical intrauterine pathology and several clarifying diagrams, a number of which were specially prepared for inclusion in this book.

A Manual of Clinical Hysteroscopy is an important contribution to the gynecological literature of our time. It presents state-of-the-art information on gynecological endoscopy together with the extensive personal experience of Dr Valle, one of the true pioneers in the field.

I believe this manual will become a classic addition to the libraries of all practicing gynecologists and gynecological surgeons. No one in this field could want a better practical reference guide than this excellent volume.

John J. Sciarra, MD, PhD
Chicago

Preface

As a self-taught hysteroscopist, over the years I have faced the many inconveniences and handicaps that usually accompany a new technique. In 1972, as a neophyte hysteroscopist, I paid a visit to Dr Rodolfo Quinones in Mexico City to observe his technique of hysteroscopy using low-viscosity fluids. Following this visit, I adapted a similar technique, using polyethylene catheters to convert the hysteroscope into a continuous-flow system. In addition, I modified the delivery system by using plastic containers that could be converted, in systems using positive pressure, by external pressure cuffs. These minor modifications assisted me in the application of low-viscosity fluids for intrauterine distention as an alternative to CO_2 gas and high-viscosity dextrans, and permitted not only distention, but also intermittent washings, particularly during operative procedures.

In 1976, as hysteroscopic clinical applications became more extensive, I began to offer a hysteroscopy workshop to gynecologists on a yearly basis. As the gynecological resectoscope and lasers were introduced, these methods were also incorporated into our clinical practice. Thus, after nearly a quarter of a century of experience in adapting methods, instrumentation and expanding clinical applications, I was rewarded with an efficient, relatively easy and effective hysteroscopy program that many physicians have subsequently adapted for themselves.

Being aware of the need for a concise, practical book on hysteroscopy with a unified philosophy, I have brought together in this volume a didactic core of diagnostic and operative hysteroscopy as a practical and concise reference volume. This manual is aimed at residents, fellows and practicing gynecologists with an interest in hysteroscopy. Although there are selected references for each chapter, it was not my intention to provide an encyclopedic bibliography.

The illustrations included in this book have been selected to show, in conjunction with the instructive 'how-to' drawings, the normal and abnormal presentations in selected instances as well as the various operative steps in selected procedures to provide the practitioner with a better understanding of the methods used. However, sound clinical medical judgment cannot be replaced by a procedure and, therefore, I have included a discussion of the indications and contraindications of hysteroscopy as well as of the management of complications, with practical guidelines for the prevention of specific complications. I hope the reader will find this to be a practical manual of the rationale and techniques for the optimal performance of various hysteroscopic procedures.

To complete the theme of uterine evaluation, there are also four chapters written by four guest contributors: Dr Alvin Siegler on hysterosalpingography; Dr Leeber Cohen on ultrasonography; Dr Frederick Hoff on computed tomography and magnetic resonance imaging; and Dr Debra Heller on uterine pathology. I am indebted to these experts for their invaluable contributions.

I am also grateful to the many colleagues who have shared their experiences and suggestions with me, in particular, Dr John J. Sciarra who, as Chairman of the Department of Obstetrics and Gynecology at Northwestern University Medical School, as well as my teacher and mentor, has sparked, and consistently encouraged and supported, my interest in hysteroscopy.

Finally, I am grateful to Parthenon Publishing for their invaluable help in making this manual a reality.

In closing, if this book provides a useful aid to physicians who are learning hysteroscopy, reassures those who are already accomplished in the procedure and improves the care provided to patients, then my goal in writing this manual will have been fulfilled.

Rafael F. Valle
Chicago

1 An introduction to hysteroscopy

Evaluation of the uterine cavity is necessary when abnormal bleeding develops and / or reproduction is impaired. Because the endometrium changes cyclically and continuously under the influence of steroids, its structure and thickness also vary and, when abnormal growth occurs, it is important to rule out those conditions that not only may be the cause of the abnormal bleeding, but may predispose the patient to malignancy. Premalignant and malignant lesions of the endometrium need to be ruled out. Other benign conditions within the uterus, such as endometrial polyps and uterine leiomyomas, may also cause abnormal bleeding and require treatment. Finally, structural developmental anomalies can occur as a result of abnormal embryogenesis, and hysteroscopy provides an excellent method of evaluation and treatment when these conditions impair reproduction.

Traditionally, the uterine cavity has been evaluated with mechanical curettes, forceps, sounds or probes, suction devices and hysterosalpingography. Whereas suction devices are useful in obtaining endometrium for histological evaluation, they may not provide accurate diagnosis of endometrial polyps and / or leiomyomas. Blind uterine exploration with curettes or forceps also lacks accuracy in evaluating the endometrial lining.

With the use of small and thin suction devices activated not by pumps, but by small plungers, endometrial evaluation becomes more difficult, particularly if the entire endometrial lining must be evaluated. These devices are most useful when the endometrium is sampled to determine the stage of maturation in infertility evaluation. When used for evaluation of abnormal uterine bleeding, however, they may not provide adequate tissue for a complete histological evaluation of the endometrial lining. Hysterosalpingography under fluoroscopic view allows evaluation of the symmetry of the uterine cavity and rules out space-occupying lesions such as polyps and / or myomas. In addition, this method provides evaluation of the Fallopian tubes, revealing their caliber, distal epithelial folds and patency. Whereas hysterosalpingography is most valuable when normal findings are obtained, additional evaluation may be necessary – should abnormal findings be encountered – to rule out false distortions simulating pathology.

Following clinical trials to establish the indications and proper place of hysteroscopy in clinical gynecology, the use of hysteroscopy expanded in the 1980s to the point where, today, it is a well-established method of evaluation and treatment of many conditions of the uterine cavity. Of late, new methods of evaluating the uterus, such as ultrasound particularly with vaginal probes, fluid-enhanced sonography and hysteroscopy, have been introduced.

Sonography allows evaluation of the uterine walls, which is not possible with endoscopic methods. The practitioner is able to rule out the presence of leiomyomas or assess their location, size and number. The endometrial lining can be evaluated and measured, particularly in postmenopausal patients who bleed abnormally.

Fluid-enhanced sonography adds another dimension to the ultrasound examination by adding contrast and permitting better evaluation of intrauterine lesions such as polyps and myomas. Because of this, the technique helps to determine the degree of penetration of these lesions into the myometrial wall, and the intramural and intraluminal components.

Hysteroscopy offers a direct view of the uterine cavity and the possibility of targeted biopsies of suspect areas. Special hysteroscopes can evaluate tissues at various magnifications, from ×20 to ×150, or at nucleocytoplasmic levels.

Recently, microendoscopes with outer diameters <3 mm were introduced to allow easier transcervical introduction and avoid anesthesia. The practical value of these endoscopes is currently being studied.

This manual reviews various aspects of diagnostic and therapeutic hysteroscopy. The current instrumentation required for diagnosis and treatment is described with practical observations regarding their use. The diagnostic and therapeutic applications of hysteroscopy, including its various indications, contraindications and possible complications, are also reviewed. The fundamental steps in the performance of diagnostic and operative hysteroscopy and resectoscopy are described with practical recommendations for simplifying the procedures.

Historical landmarks in the development of hysteroscopy

The major historical landmarks in the development of hysteroscopy are summarized in Table 1.1. In 1807, Phillip Bozzini developed the first known endoscope to view the interior of the uterus and / or

urinary bladder (Figure 1.1). In 1853, Antonin Désormeaux presented a model of the first truly workable cystoscope (Figure 1.2) to the French Academy of Medicine. This scope had a reflecting mirror with a central perforation for viewing. However, it was not until 1869 that Pantaleoni used a modified endoscope in a clinical setting to evaluate the uterine cavity in a postmenopausal patient complaining of abnormal uterine bleeding. Polyps were found and cauterized with silver nitrate, using the endoscope as a guide.

The first practical contact endoscope was introduced by David in 1905. This endoscope had a distal lens that permitted

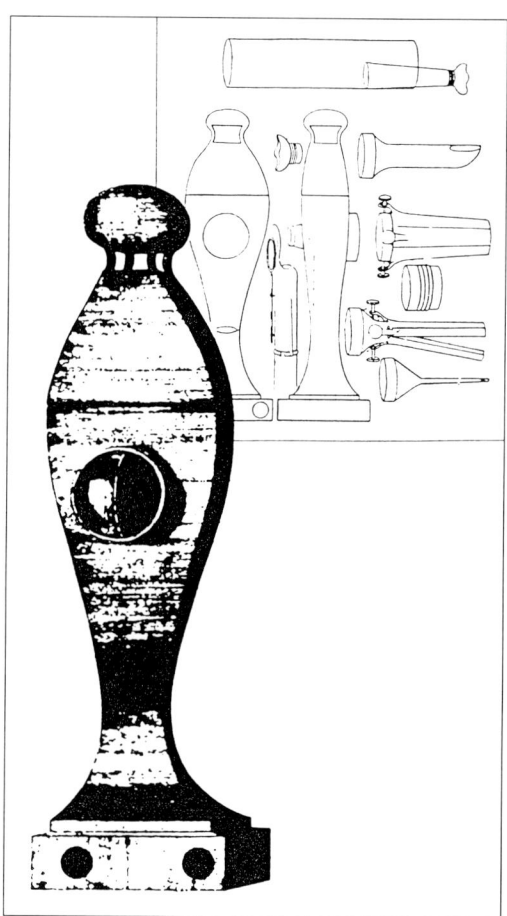

Figure 1.1 Bozzini's light conductor, devised in the early 1800s, was a candlelit specular instrument for illumination of body cavities

Table 1.1 Milestones in the development of hysteroscopy

Year	Investigator	Contribution
1807	Bozzini	First endoscope (light conductor)
1869	Pantaleoni	First hysteroscopic examination in living patient
1879	Nitze	Cystoscope with distal illumination
1907	David	First contact hysteroscope
1914	Heineberg	System for irrigating uterine cavity
1925	Rubin	CO_2 for uterine distention
1926	Seymour	Hysteroscope with inflow and outflow channels
1927	Mikulicz-Radecki & Fruend	Biopsy-taking capability, cornual electrocoagulation
1928	Gauss	Intrauterine photography
1934	Schroeder	Measurement of intrauterine pressures
1934–1943	Segond	Irrigating system and biopsies
1936	Schack	Identified applications
1942–1970	Norment	Rubber balloon, practical irrigating system, cutting loop, fiberoptics
1953–1978	Mohri & Mohri	Fiberhysteroscope for intrauterine visualization tubaloscopy
1957	Englund *et al.*	Evaluation of abnormal uterine bleeding comparing hysterography and dilatation and curettage with hysteroscopy
1962	Silander	Studied endometrial carcinoma using silastic balloon
1968	Menken	Tubal cannulation, polyvinylpyrrolidone
1970	Edstrom & Fernstrom	32% dextran
1972	Quinones *et al.*	Tubal catheterization applications
1974	Edstrom	Therapeutic applications
1974	Parent *et al.*	Contact hysteroscopy
1978	Neuwirth	Use of resectoscope
1980	Hamou	Microhysteroscope
1981	Goldrath *et al.*	Laser endometrial ablation

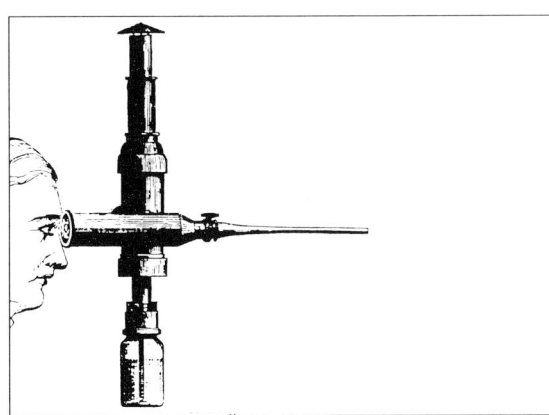 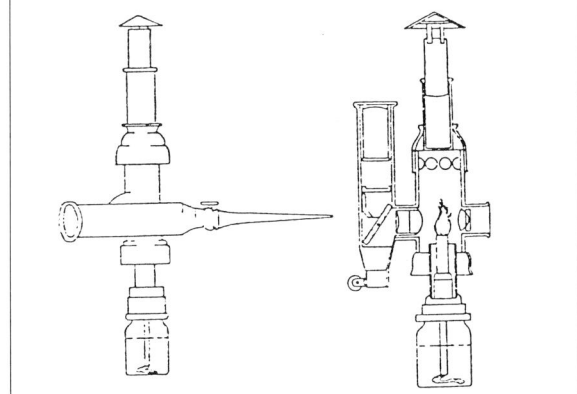

Figure 1.2 Désormeaux's first workable endoscope (left), as presented to the French Academy of Medicine in 1853, comprised a jar at the bottom holding alcohol, with a wick that extended into the central part of the instrument (middle). A cutaway view (right) shows that the flame in the central part of the instrument had a reflecting mirror to the right and a lens to the left

visualization of uterine lesions on contact. No distending medium was necessary and external light was introduced into the uterus by reflection. Heineberg in 1914 and Seymour in 1935 advanced the possibilities of continuous flow systems to look into the uterus. Practical methods using low-viscosity fluids to distend the uterus were introduced by Norment in 1950, followed in 1958 by the application of the first rudimentary gynecological resectoscope with a loop electrode to remove myomas and polyps. In the late 1960s, Menken developed a special hysteroscope designed for tubal cannulation (Figure 1.3), using a high-viscosity mixture of linear polymers of different chain lengths and molecular weights, or polyvinylpirrolidone, allowing passage of catheters into the tubal ostium.

In 1970, Edstrom and Fernstrom introduced a method of hysteroscopy using a high-viscosity dextran (Hyskon®) that improved visualization and permitted intrauterine surgery. Lindemann perfected the delivery of CO_2 gas as a distending medium for hysteroscopy, with special machines designed to calibrate the flow and intrauterine pressure produced by the gas. In 1974, the initial therapeutic applications of hysteroscopy were established by Edstrom,

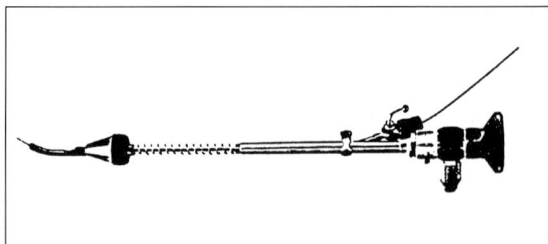

Figure 1.3 The hysteroscope devised by Menken in the late 1960s for tubal cannulation

including the division of intrauterine adhesions, treatment of uterine septa and resection of submucous leiomyomas.

In 1980, a microcolpohysteroscope was introduced by Hamou. This instrument permitted magnification of tissue at different degrees – ×20, ×60 and ×150 – or at nucleocytoplasmic levels. The Nd:YAG laser was approved by the US Food and Drug Administration as a tool to perform endometrial ablation in 1986, and the resectoscope was approved for gynecological procedures in 1989. In the late 1980s, a high-resolution, high-sensitivity, light videocamera was specifically designed for endoscopy.

While the technology continues to develop, the improvements in instrumentation and ancillary equipment have kept pace with the use and applications of hysteroscopy as a diagnostic and therapeutic tool.

Selected bibliography

Bush RB, Leonhardt H, Bush IM, Lands RR. Dr. Bozzini's Lichleiter. A translation of his original article (1806). *Urology* 1974;3:119

Harrison RM. The development of modern endoscopy. *J Med Primatol* 1976;5:73

Lindemann HJ. Historical aspects of hysteroscopy. *Fertil Steril* 1973;24:230

Norment WB. The hysteroscope. *Am J Obstet Gynecol* 1956;71:426

Pearlman SJ. Bozzini's classical treatise on endoscopy: A translation. *Quart Bull Northwest Univ Med School* 1949;23:332

Rathert P, Lutzeyer W, Goddwin WE. Philip Bozzini (1773–1809) and the Lichtleiter. *Urology* 1974;3:113

Valle RF. Hysteroscopy. In Wynn RM, ed. *Obstetrics and Gynecology Annual*, Vol. 7. New York: Appleton-Century-Crofts, 1978:245–83

Valle RF, Sciarra JJ. Current status of hysteroscopy in gynecologic practice. *Fertil Steril* 1979;32:619

2 General principles and instrumentation

The basic requirements for the performance of hysteroscopy include an endoscope or hysteroscope, media to distend the cavity of the uterus, and an appropriate light source to transmit adequate illumination via fiberoptic cables.

Although the first known endoscope to observe hollow organs, such as the urinary bladder and the uterus, was introduced by Bozzini in 1807, the practical clinical applications of endoscopy to visualize the uterine cavity did not occur until the late 1960s and early 1970s, with the introduction of endoscopes specifically designed to visualize this organ. The most cumbersome impediment to the use of hysteroscopy in a clinical setting was solved with the availability of safe and effective media to distend the uterine cavity. Fiberoptics has greatly improved visualization by illuminating this small cavity that is surrounded by thick muscular layers.

The hysteroscope

There are two types of hysteroscope – rigid and flexible. Modern rigid hysteroscopes are of two kinds – diagnostic and operative.

Diagnostic hysteroscopes

These are in general no larger than 4 mm in outer diameter and permit uterine distention by delivering CO_2 gas (Figure 2.1). Because of their size, these hysteroscopes do not provide an operative channel. The telescope has either a straightforward 0° angle of view or a 30° foreoblique view, which is most

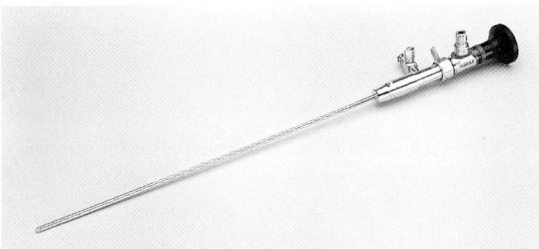

Figure 2.1 Diagnostic hysteroscope with a 10.5-F (2.7-mm) sheath

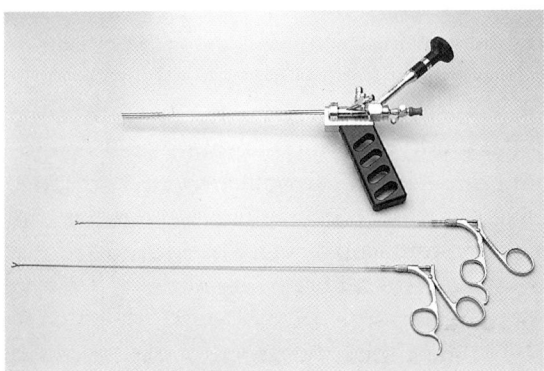

Figure 2.2 Compact hysteroscope (15-F diameter) with handle (upper), and 5-F semirigid forceps and grasper (middle and lower)

commonly used to visualize the uterotubal junctions. There are other diagnostic hysteroscopes with slightly larger outer diameters of 5–6 mm, with distal fenestrations that permit continuous flow when low-viscosity fluids are used to distend the uterus. Although these hysteroscopes may also have small operating channels, only mild conditions can be treated, and biopsies taken with small-caliber forceps are generally inadequate for proper histological evaluation (Figures 2.2 and 2.3).

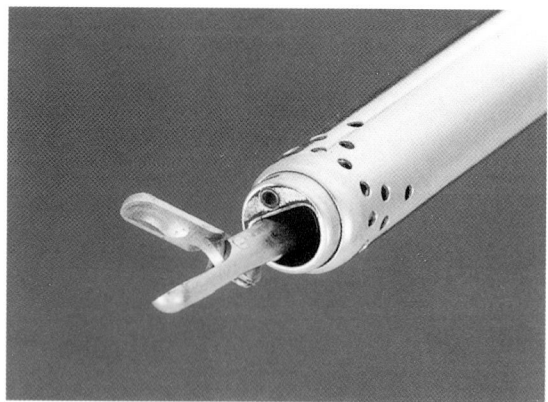

Figure 2.3 Close-up view of distal tip of a diagnostic–operative hysteroscope with a continuous-flow outer sheath and flexible forceps in the operating channel

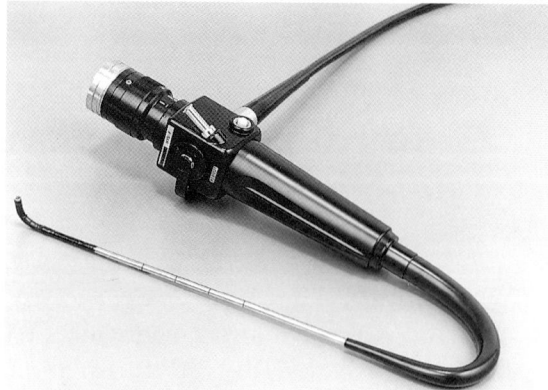

Figure 2.4 Flexible diagnostic hysteroscope (3.5-mm outer diameter)

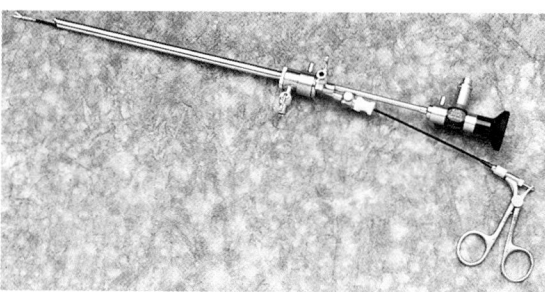

Figure 2.5 Operative hysteroscope (7-mm outer diameter) with flexible forceps in place

Other diagnostic hysteroscopes may have the capability of magnification, such as the Hamou hysteroscope or microcolpohysteroscope, with an additional offside ocular that can increase the magnification twenty-fold for a panoramic view, or to $\times 60$ or $\times 150$ for a contact view. The latter magnification can evaluate tissues at the nucleocytoplasmic level. The instrument can also be used for evaluation of the ectocervix on contact.

While smaller-caliber endoscopes of <3 mm in diameter have been used as diagnostic hysteroscopes, their size permits neither a clear view nor similar resolution to telescopes that are 3–4 mm in diameter. When the telescope decreases in size, the field of view is reduced and, despite the use of high-sensitivity light cameras, the video projection of the image is diminished.

The flexible diagnostic hysteroscopes, usually 3.5 mm in outer diameter, are excellent alternatives for diagnosis (Figure 2.4). In addition to their distal steerability, they have an additional feature that allows the tip to be bent according to need. This can be helpful in markedly anteflexed or retroflexed uteri in guiding the instrument

atraumatically towards the uterine cavity. When pathology such as tumors that distort the symmetry of the uterine cavity or intrauterine adhesions is present, the steerability of this instrument helps in the guided introduction and exploration of the uterus. With these flexible diagnostic hysteroscopes, either CO_2 gas or low-viscosity fluids can be used as distending media.

Operative hysteroscopes

These hysteroscopes have telescopes 4 mm in outer diameter and require a larger operative sheath, usually 7–8 mm in outer diameter, and an operative channel to permit 7-F instruments, either flexible or semirigid, to be inserted and manipulated (Figure 2.5). Most modern operative hysteroscopes have

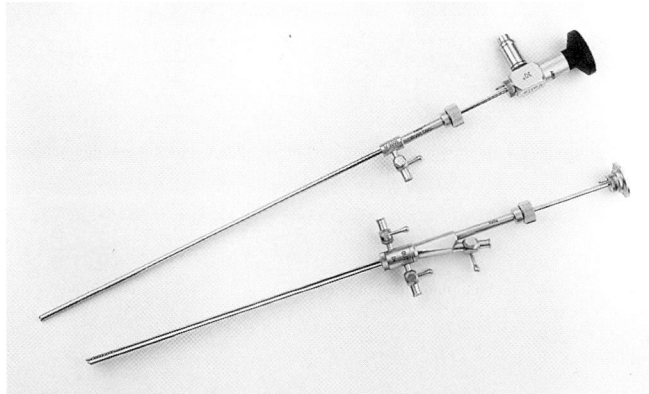

Figure 2.6 Diagnostic-operative hysteroscope with (lower) and without (upper) continuous-flow outer sheath

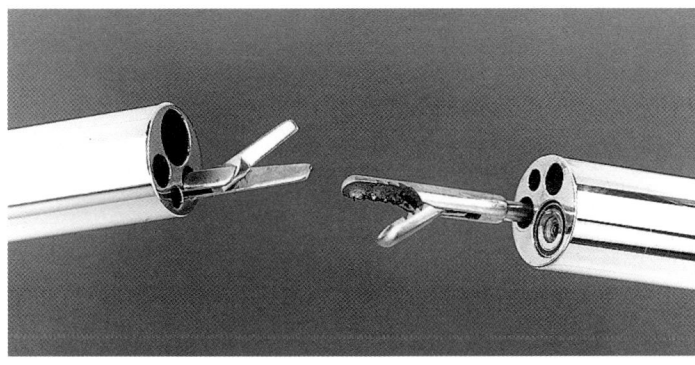

Figure 2.7 Double-channel operating hysteroscope with ancillary instruments in place

some type of continuous flow system to permit washing of the uterine cavity (Figure 2.6), but because this washing effect is not as efficient as that provided by the resectoscope when targeted areas need to be cleansed of blood clots or debris, a polyethylene catheter is inserted in the operating channel to perform this specific function. Recently, outer sheaths with distal fenestrations have been used to permit retrieval and collection of fluid, and continuous lavage of the uterine cavity.

New hysteroscopes with more than one operating channel have been designed to permit not only continuous flow, but additional means of surgical manipulation in the uterine cavity. The outer diameter of these instruments can be increased to 8–9 mm, so these instruments require cervical dilatation of 9.5–10 mm (Figure 2.7).

Flexible operative hysteroscopes are also available with an outer diameter of

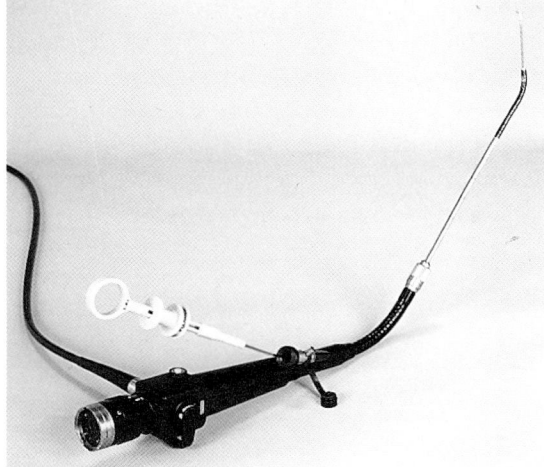

Figure 2.8 Flexible operative hysteroscope (4.9-mm diameter) with flexible forceps in place

4.9 mm and an operating channel with an inner diameter of 2.5 mm for instrumentation (Figure 2.8). Flexible operative hysteroscopes permit the introduction of significantly smaller instruments than permitted with rigid instrumentation without significant cervical dilatation, thereby decreasing trauma. Because of their capability for flexing the distal tip, they are excellent alternatives for tubal cannulation, permitting catheters to be placed in the direction of the tubal opening. This is particularly useful in patients with laterally recessed tubal cornual junctions and in those who have T-shaped uterine cavities. Fiberoptic lasers can be guided more easily through flexible hysteroscopes, should they be required for treatment of lesions at the cornua or for laterally placed lesions in the uterine walls such as intrauterine adhesions.

Ancillary instruments

To perform hysteroscopic surgery, several instruments may be required, such as scissors, grasping forceps, biopsy forceps, catheters and electroprobes. These instruments are usually 7 F in diameter and fit snugly in the operating channel. The most commonly used ancillary operative instruments are the semirigid type (Figure 2.9) that can be bent somewhat and inserted into the operating channel with ease, targeting the area without much manipulation of the hysteroscope itself. Alternatively, there are other forceps designed for operative hysteroscopy that can

be used when sturdier instruments are required – the so-called optical forceps or optical scissors (Figure 2.10). These are assembled in the hysteroscope and cannot be moved unless the whole hysteroscope is moved. While these rigid instruments perform better when cutting, grasping or during biopsy, care should be taken to control their action at all times under panoramic view and to introduce them only under direct vision. The panoramic view of the uterine cavity may be impaired as they are fixed to the end of the endoscope and cannot be moved independently. These rigid optical instruments should be used selectively and only in special situations (Figures 2.11 and 2.12).

While most operative procedures with a hysteroscope are performed with flexible or semirigid instrumentation, electroprobes can also be used to coagulate or divide tissues. Differently shaped electroprobes are available (Figure 2.13) and their use requires the same precautions as when using electricity in any other part of the body.

Light sources

Most light sources are the halogen type of 300–400 W. When video systems are used, it

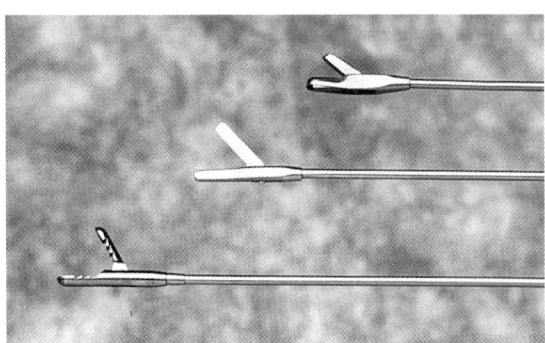

Figure 2.9 Semirigid ancillary hysteroscopic instruments (7-F diameter) include, from upper to lower, biopsy forceps, scissors and grasping forceps

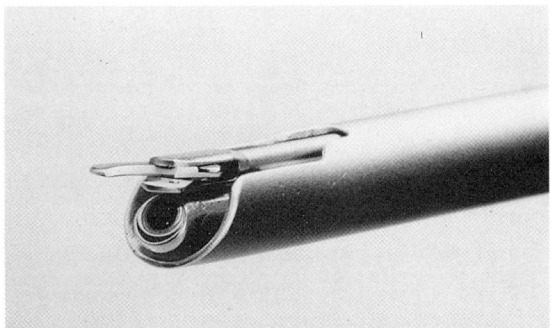

Figure 2.10 Sturdy optical scissors fixed at the distal end of a hysteroscope

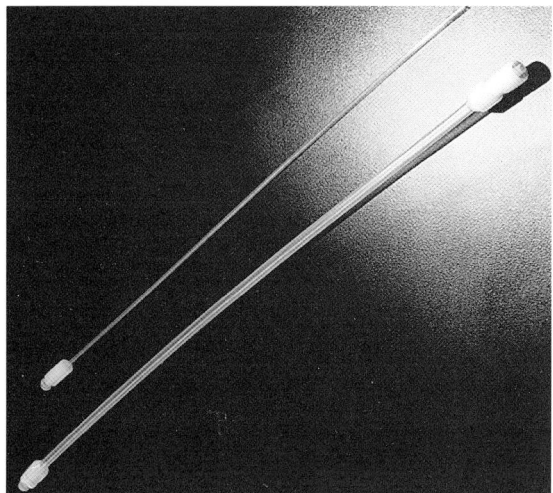

Figure 2.11 Plastic cannulas can be used for intrauterine flushing (right) or instillation of high-viscosity fluid (left)

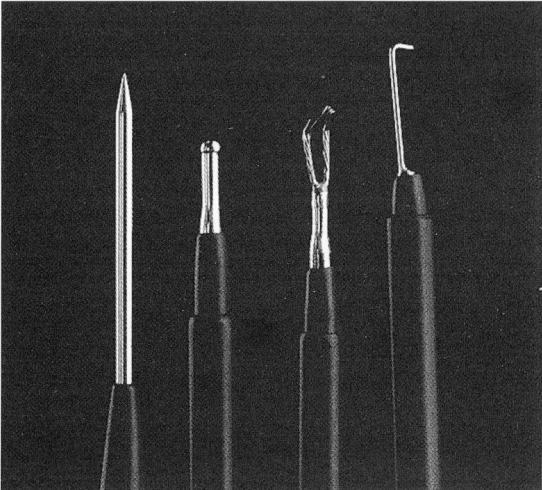

Figure 2.13 Ancillary electrode tips for hysteroscopy are available in various configurations (left to right): needle; ball; loop; and hook

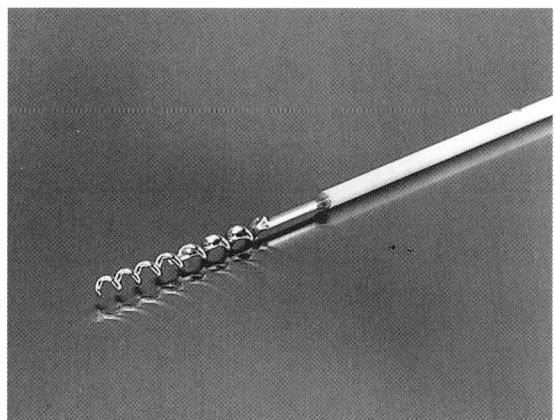

Figure 2.12 Hysteroscopic corkscrew (7-F diameter) for myoma stabilization and removal

is important to have a light source that can provide adequate illumination to obtain the best resolution. Ideally, xenon or a halide light source should be used. Nonetheless, with the new high-sensitivity light cameras (3-chip cameras), the need for powerful light sources has markedly decreased. It is important, however, to replace the fiberoptic cables transmitting the light when breakage of fibers is observed by illuminating a surface directly with a light-transmitting cable.

Basic instrumentation in hysteroscopy

Not many instruments are required for hysteroscopy, but it is important to have the correct instruments available during an examination.

For diagnostic hysteroscopy, a telescope and a diagnostic sheath with a diameter <4 mm are necessary as well as plastic tubing to conduct the CO_2 gas, a fiberoptic light-transmitting cable, a vaginal speculum to visualize the cervix, soft sponges for disinfection, a tonsil needle with an appropriate syringe to perform a paracervical block and a long tenaculum to stabilize the cervix.

Operative hysteroscopy requires a telescope 4 mm in outer diameter, a hysteroscopic bridge with a sheath 7–8 mm in outer diameter, plastic nipples to occlude the inner and outer ports, semirigid instrumentation including scissors, biopsy forceps and grasping forceps, and soft polyethylene catheters with an inner diameter of 1.67 mm and an outer diameter of 2.42 mm to permit selective cleansing of the uterine cavity. A videocamera recorder is most useful during diagnostic hysteroscopy, and is necessary during operative hysteroscopy not only for documentation, but also because it permits an easier and more comfortable operation for the endoscopist. In addition, it provides excellent magnification and resolution of various tissues, enhancing the ease and precision of the procedure, and allows the assisting team to observe and assist with the operation.

Cleansing and maintenance of instruments

After use, the endoscopes, hysteroscopes and resectoscopes and their components should be thoroughly rinsed and washed with special brushes and soaps. The ports and channels should be delicately cleaned with soft wire brushes and rinsed appropriately.

Disinfection and sterilization

While most instruments can be disinfected with solutions such as glutaraldehyde (Cidex®), overnight gas sterilization is the most commonly used method to safely sterilize and maintain the instruments ready for use. An autoclave can be used for all metallic parts except the telescope, plastic nipples and flexible plastic-coated instruments. The flexible hysteroscope needs cleaning, disinfection and sterilization with gas only. During storage, it is important to avoid dropping, bumping or bending these delicate instruments. The telescope should be kept in a separate container to avoid breakage.

Selected bibliography

Baggish MS. A new laser hysteroscope for Nd-YAG endometrial ablation. *Laser Surg Med* 1988;8:248

Brueschke EE, Wilbanks GD. A steerable fiberoptic hysteroscope. *Obstet Gynecol* 1974; 44:273

Garner FM. Optical physics with emphasis on endoscopes. In Baggish MS, ed. *Gynecologic Endoscopy and Instrumentation, Vol. 26. Clinical Obstetrics and Gynecology*. Hagerstown, MD: Harper & Row, 1983:213–8

Hamou J. Microhysteroscopy. A new procedure and its original applications in gynecology. *J Reprod Med* 1981;26:375

Hopkins HH. Optical principles of the endoscope. In Berti G, ed. *Endoscopy*. New York: Appleton-Century-Crofts, 1976:3–26

Iglesias JJ, Sporer A, Gellman AC, Seebode JJ. New Iglesias resectoscope with continuous irrigation, simultaneous suction, and low intravesicle pressure. *J Urol* 1975;114:929

Lin BL, Miyamoto N, Tomatsu M, *et al.* Flexible hysterofiberscope. The development of a new flexible hysterofiberscope and its clinical applications. *Acta Obstet Gynaecol Jpn* 1987; 39:649

McCarthy JF. A new type observation and operating cystourethroscope. *J Urol* 1923;10:519

Parent B, Guedj H, Barbot J, Nodarian P. *Panoramic Hysteroscopy*. (English translation). Baltimore, MD: Williams & Wilkins, 1987

Prescott R. Optical principles of endoscopy. *J Med Primatol* 1976;5:133

Quint RH. The rigid hysteroscope. In Sciarra JJ, Butler JC, Speidel JJ, eds. *Hysteroscopic Sterilization*. New York: Intercontinental Medical Book Corporation, 1974:11–18

Valle RF, Sciarra JJ. Current status of hysteroscopy in gynecologic practice. *Fertil Steril* 1979; 32:619

Valle RF. Hysteroscopy for gynecologic diagnosis. In Baggish MS, ed. *Gynecologic Endoscopy and Instrumentation, Vol. 26. Clinical Obstetrics and Gynecology*. Hagerstown, MD: Harper & Row, 1983:253–76

Valle RF. Future growth and development of hysteroscopy. In DeCherney AH, ed. *Hysteroscopy, Obstetrics and Gynecology Clinics of North America*. Philadelphia, PA: WB Saunders, 1988:111–26

3 Uterine distention: Media and techniques

For panoramic hysteroscopy, the uterine walls that are normally in apposition must be distended to create a true cavity (Table 3.1). The urinary bladder can easily be distended with gravity pressure. The thin distensible walls and epithelial lining do not change cyclically. As it is lined with a simple cuboidal epithelium, the bladder is an ideal organ for distention during cystoscopy. Furthermore, the urinary bladder has a much greater capacity than the uterus, and there is no communication between the bladder and the peritoneal cavity. For these reasons, cystoscopy can easily be performed without special equipment to distend the bladder.

In contrast, the uterus has thick muscular walls that require positive pressure for its distention. The uterine lining comprises cylindrical columnar epithelium that changes with each monthly cycle; the thickness, consistency, structure and vascularization make the performance of hysteroscopy particularly cumbersome in the luteal phase. The uterine cavity communicates directly with the peritoneal cavity, should fluid enter the Fallopian tubes. It is important, therefore, to understand the possible sequelae and pay attention to details when converting this potential cavity into an actual one. This is why hysteroscopy took longer than cystoscopy to become established as a practical technique.

Media for uterine distention

Three different types of media can be used safely and effectively to distend the uterus: CO_2 gas; low-viscosity fluids; and high-viscosity fluids.

CO_2 gas

The use of CO_2 gas requires electronic monitoring of the intrauterine gas pressure and the rate at which the gas is delivered (Figure 3.1). CO_2 gas is highly diffusible and soluble, permitting the continuous elimination of small quantities of intravasated gas by the lungs, using the enormous buffer capacity of the blood circulation as gas is

Table 3.1 Factors related to panoramic endoscopy of the uterus and urinary bladder

Uterus	Urinary bladder
Virtual cavity with thick muscle walls	Thin muscle walls are easily distensible
Positive pressure needed for distention	Distensible with only gravity pressure
Bleeds at monthly cycles	No cylical bleeding
Has columnar epithelium with glands	Has transitional epithelium
Epithelium changes cyclically	No cyclical changes
Communicates with peritoneal cavity via Fallopian tubes	No communication with peritoneal cavity
Has individual embryology, anatomy, physiology and and pathology	Has different embryology, anatomy, physiology and and pathology

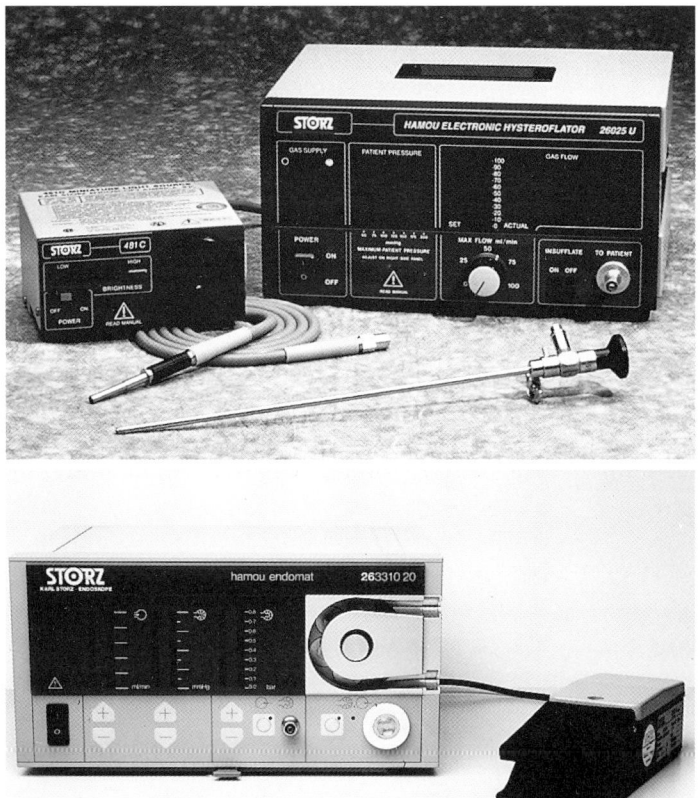

Figure 3.1 An electronic hysterosufflator for uterine distention with CO_2 gas (upper); and an electronic pump for uterine distention with low-viscosity fluid (lower)

continuously intravasated. With excessive amounts of intravasation, particularly if excessively high flow rates are used and if the intrauterine pressure markedly exceeds the mean arterial pressure, decompensation may occur. Therefore, it is important to use machines specifically designed for hysteroscopy which can calibrate not only the flow of the gas to around 40–50 mL / min, but also intrauterine pressure (not to exceed 150 mmHg). Most hysteroscopic examinations can be performed at a flow rate of approximately 30–40 mL / min with an intrauterine pressure at approximately 60–70 mmHg. These two parameters compensate each other to maintain a proper balance. When the intrauterine pressure increases, the flow rate decreases, and *vice versa*.

CO_2 gas insufflation has several advantages. It is a 'clean' medium, permitting excellent visualization as there is no interposition of a substance to cause refraction, and adequately maintains distention of the uterine cavity. Nonetheless, there are some disadvantages particularly when used for operative procedures. If CO_2 gas is mixed with blood, it may produce bubbling, which is cumbersome and may obscure the view. Because CO_2 gas is invisible, a leak in the system may not be noticed for some time. A specific machine is required for electronic calibration of the CO_2 flow rate and pressure. Finally, use of a laser becomes cumbersome due to the smoke and fumes that cannot be easily evacuated without deflating the uterine cavity. However, it remains the best choice for diagnostic hysteroscopy as it uses small hysteroscopes <4 mm in outer diameter that do not require cervical dilatation.

Low-viscosity fluids

Low-viscosity fluids are useful during operative procedures as they permit not only washing of the uterine cavity, but also lavage of the blood clots and debris that may form during an operation. These fluids are of two types: those containing electrolytes; and those that do not. Low-viscosity fluids containing electrolytes, specifically sodium in the form of sodium chloride (NaCl), are used when operative procedures are performed with mechanical tools or lasers that require no electricity. The presence of electrolytes makes the procedure somewhat safer and prevents hyponatremia, should excessive amounts of fluid be used and absorbed. The quantity of fluid used should be carefully monitored, with measurement of the amount of fluid instilled and recovered to permit estimation of the amount of fluid absorbed by the patient (Figure 3.2).

The most commonly used electrolyte-containing fluids for uterine distention are normal saline (0.9% NaCl), dextrose 5% in 50% saline (0.45% NaCl) and Ringer's lactate solution. All are equally effective in distending the uterine cavity and providing good visualization. Because these fluids are usually packaged in plastic bags containing 1000 mL, some positive pressure is necessary to distend the uterus adequately as gravity pressure is not sufficient under these circumstances. Alternatively, a mechanical pump such as those that measure fluid pressure and flow rate can be used, limiting the intrauterine pressure to no more than 100–120 mmHg. Nonetheless, even with such pumps, special care should be taken to monitor inflow and outflow to estimate the amount of unrecovered fluid.

Low-viscosity fluids without electrolytes are required during electrosurgery with either the hysteroscope or resectoscope. Electrolytes are excellent conductors, but may disperse the electrical output erratically so that the desired effect on tissues may not be safely obtained. These fluids include dextrose 5% in water, glycine 1.5%, sorbitol 3%, a combination of sorbitol 2.8% and mannitol 0.5% and, finally, a mannitol 5% solution. Despite some differences in the osmolality of these substances, for practical purposes and for visualization, there are no major differences. Ideally, the solution should not change either plasma osmolality or plasma electrolytes; because these fluids contain no electrolytes, hyponatremia may occur if excessive amounts are absorbed by the patient. Mannitol 5%, an osmotic diuretic, decreases this risk; nonetheless, in the acute state, sodium may be lost and, therefore, careful monitoring of these patients is required.

Most of these substances, particularly glycine and sorbitol, are packaged in 3-L plastic containers. If large-bore or urological tubing is used, and the bags are elevated above the patient to approximately 80 cm, then enough pressure is obtained to deliver these fluids by gravity alone, permitting adequate distention of the uterine cavity without the need for tourniquets or pumps. To obtain this effect, which is feasible with all resectoscopes, only hysteroscopes with continuous flow systems are appropriate.

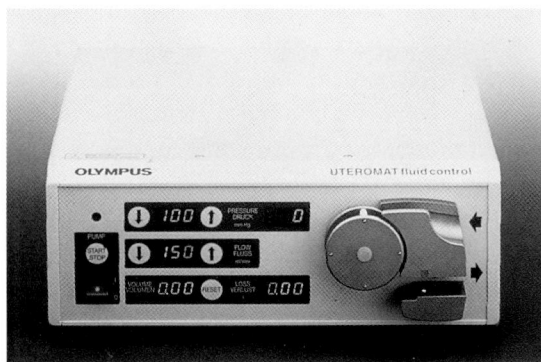

Figure 3.2 Automatic pump for optimal fluid control

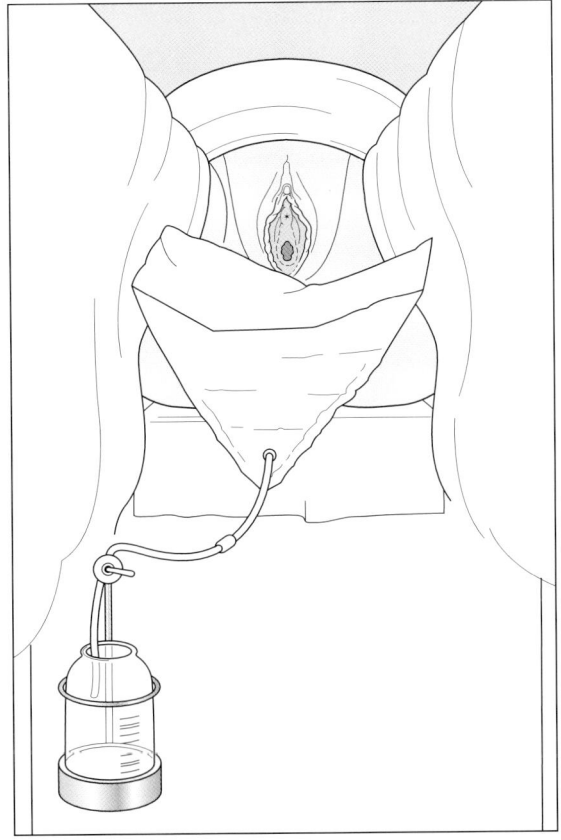

Figure 3.3 Pouch for collecting fluid

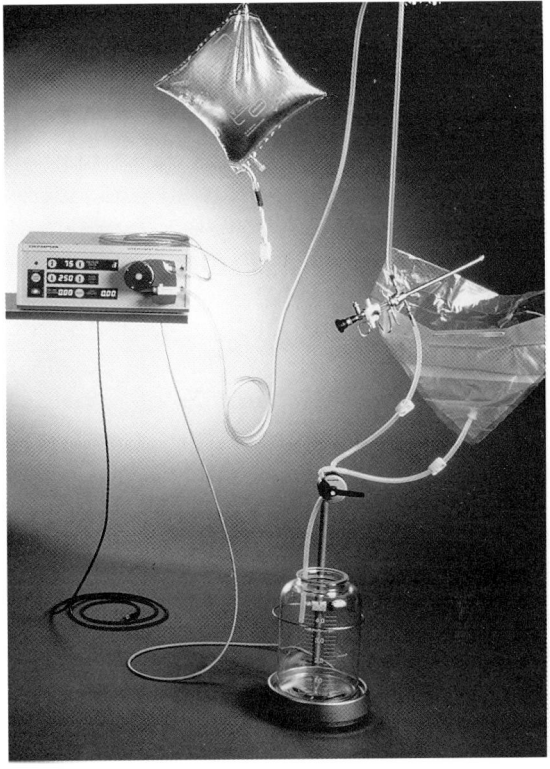

Figure 3.4 Fluid management system with an electronic pump for use in an office or operating suite

Low-viscosity fluids offer several advantages. They can clear debris, mucus and blood clots from the operative field and continuously wash the uterine cavity, permitting good visualization. Should the mechanism be faulty and leakage of fluid occur, it will be immediately visible, and the fluid instilled and recovered can easily be measured. Because these fluids, particularly those without electrolytes, may be intravasated, care should be taken to monitor meticulously the amount of fluid not recovered to alert the practitioner of intravasation and absorption by the patient. Although low-viscosity fluids may cross the Fallopian tubes, in general, the amount needed to distend the uterus is small and should not cause

serious problems in the patient. In addition, when fluids without electrolytes are used, fluid deficits should be carefully monitored in view of the possibility of hyponatremia when excessive absorption occurs.

Ancillary equipment to monitor recovery of low-viscosity fluids

Plastic pouches can be modified and added to drapes or attached to the patient to permit adequate collection of fluid (Figure 3.3). These pouches are attached to special suction machines via large-port tubes that permit accurate recovery of this fluid into calibrated containers to measure the total outflow (Figure 3.4).

High-viscosity fluids

The most commonly used high-viscosity fluid is dextran with a high molecular weight (MW) – 70 000 MW – in a 10% water solution. This medium is highly viscous and, therefore, only small amounts are usually required for an examination as the flow is slow on entering or exiting the uterine cavity. Dextran provides excellent visualization due to its high refractory index and offers an excellent alternative to distention of the uterus when bleeding occurs in the uterine cavity, as it does not mix with blood. Usually, examination can be performed despite a small amount of bleeding. Because dextran is a hyperosmotic solution, intravasation of excessive amounts may precipitate serious effects such as pulmonary edema of non-cardiogenic origin and even coagulopathies due to changes produced in the cascade of coagulation factors.

Although it is evident that some type of mechanical pump is necessary to deliver these fluids safely and effectively, as yet, there is no such pump that is practical, totally safe and inexpensive. Specific intra-uterine transducers are necessary for adequate measurement of intrauterine pressure, flow rate, and the amounts of fluid injected, recovered and potentially absorbed by the patient.

Techniques for uterine distention

Panoramic hysteroscopy

For diagnostic or operative hysteroscopy, the patient is placed on an appropriate table in a dorsal lithotomy position. A bimanual pelvic examination is performed to assess uterine size and direction. After proper disinfection of the vagina and vulva, a vaginal speculum is put into position and a paracervical block performed, if necessary. The anterior lip of the cervix is grasped with a single-tooth tenaculum. When using a diagnostic hysteroscope, the endoscope attached to its light source and the CO_2 gas distending medium is introduced at the level of the ectocervix

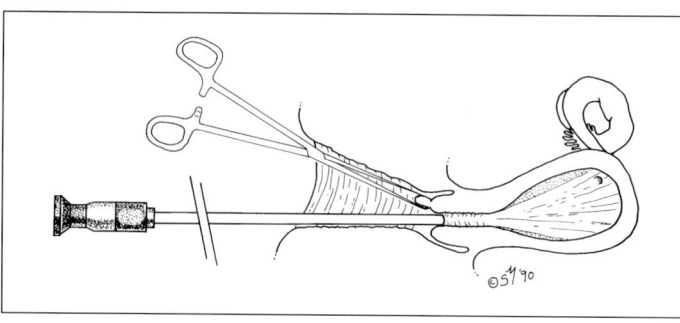

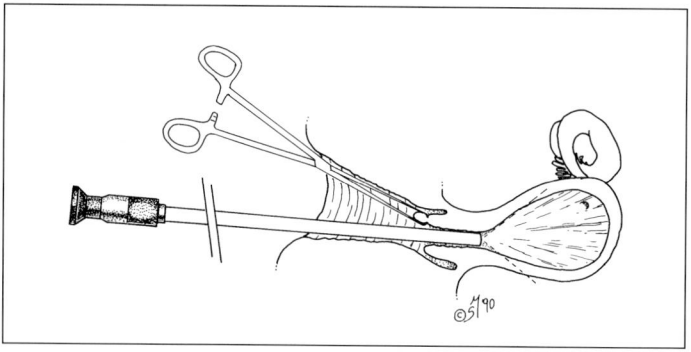

Figure 3.5 Position of a diagnostic endoscope (upper; 4 mm in outer diameter) compared with an operative hysteroscope (lower; >6 mm in outer diameter) for examination

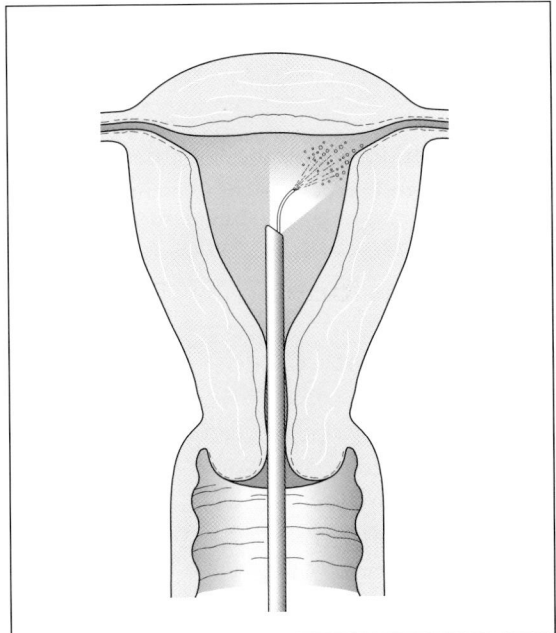

Figure 3.6 Flushing the uterine cavity using a polyethylene catheter inserted through the operative channel of a hysteroscope

before performing the systematic examination (Figure 3.5).

CO$_2$ gas hysteroscopy

When using CO$_2$ gas, it is important to check and calibrate the hysterosufflator machine that delivers the CO$_2$ gas to ensure that there is an adequate reserve of gas and that the machine is working properly. A plastic tube is attached to the hysteroscope and, with the stop-cock open, the flow rate is monitored. Gas pressure is recorded by the machine on opening and closing of the stop-cock.

Hysteroscopy with low-viscosity fluids

With low-viscosity fluids, only hysteroscopes that permit continuous flow should be used. Before distention of the uterus, the uterine cavity should be cleared of debris, blood clots and mucus by inserting a polyethylene

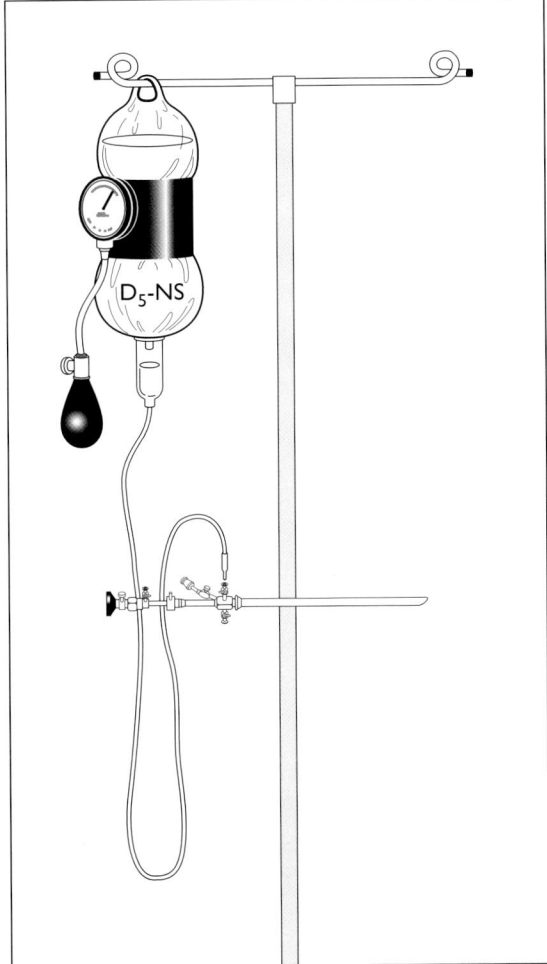

Figure 3.7 Instillation of fluids into the uterus using a plastic bag with a pressure cuff

catheter through the operative channel (Figure 3.6). Such cleansing is important because most procedures performed with low-viscosity fluids are operative procedures using hysteroscopes which are 7–8 mm in outer diameter and almost always require cervical dilatation. If smaller diagnostic hysteroscopes with continuous-flow systems are used, then the continuous-flow system of the hysteroscope may be sufficient to cleanse the uterine cavity. Once the uterine cavity has been cleansed and the fluid retrieved through the polyethylene catheter is clear, uterine distention can begin (Figure 3.7).

Hysteroscopy with high-viscosity fluids

When using high-viscosity fluids such as dextran, it is important to reload the 50-mL syringes with the fluid and to prime the tubes by injecting the fluid until it appears at the end of the syringe. Once the tube is attached to the hysteroscope, an assistant may slowly press on the plunger of the syringe until the uterus distends. The hysteroscopist may ask the assistant to increase the pressure as necessary, depending on the examination and visualization. It is important with high-viscosity fluids to wash the instruments immediately after their use to prevent caramelization or hardening of the dextran around the instrument as this may 'freeze' the stop-cocks and locks of the instruments, making them inoperable.

Practical considerations for technique and examination

Most telescopes have a foreoblique view (25–30°; Figure 3.8). The standard position of the hysteroscope is with the light cord facing downwards so that the direction of view is upwards; thus, the anterior wall of the cervix is seen more clearly than the posterior wall (Figure 3.9). The resectoscope has the light cord facing upwards so that the direction of view is somewhat downwards to observe the fitted electroprobe.

To introduce the scope, a slow side-to-side motion can be used and, once the uterine cavity is reached, this rotational motion can be increased in a clockwise or counterclockwise direction to observe the cornual regions and tubal openings. This rotational motion is not necessary with flexible endoscopes which compensate for the foreoblique view by allowing the tip of the instrument to be steered or bent towards the area under observation. Flexible hysteroscopes are

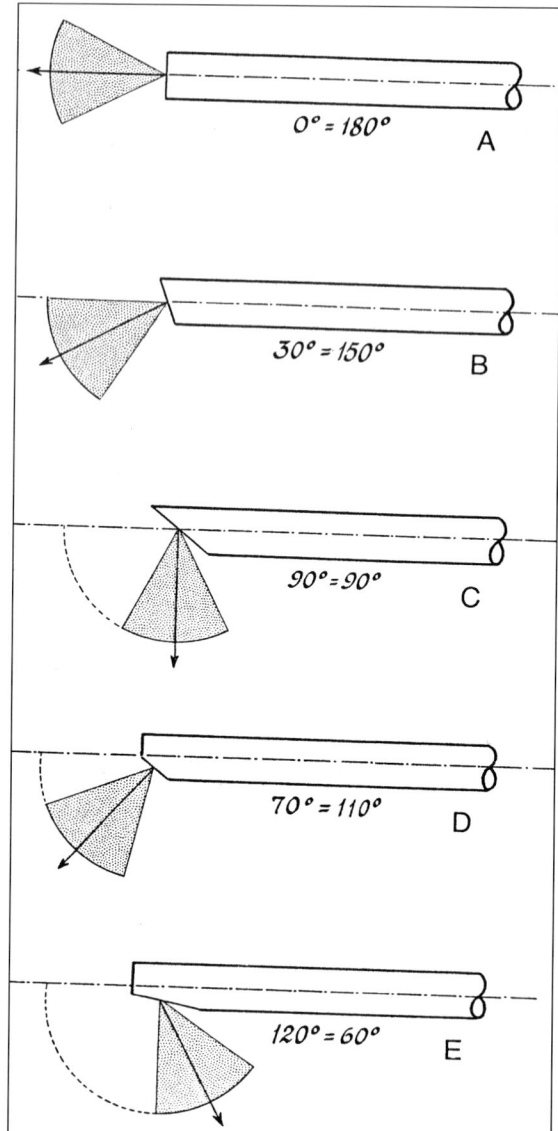

Figure 3.8 The direction and angle of view changes with the shape (angle) of the distal lens

introduced with the distal tip pointing straight ahead and are bent only while in the uterine cavity, or when entering a markedly anteflexed or retroflexed uterus. If a myoma or adhesion interferes with the panoramic view of the uterine cavity or with the initial introduction, these instruments can be driven in by bending the distal tip to accommodate the endoscope to the particular distortion.

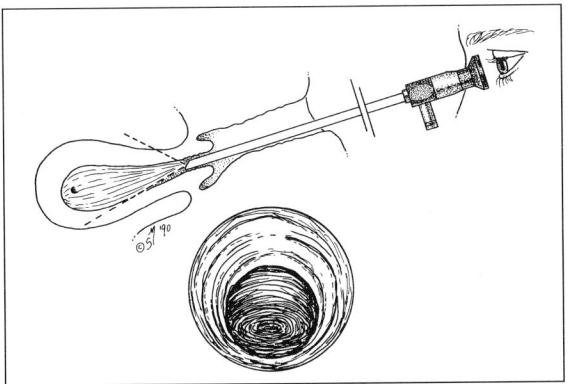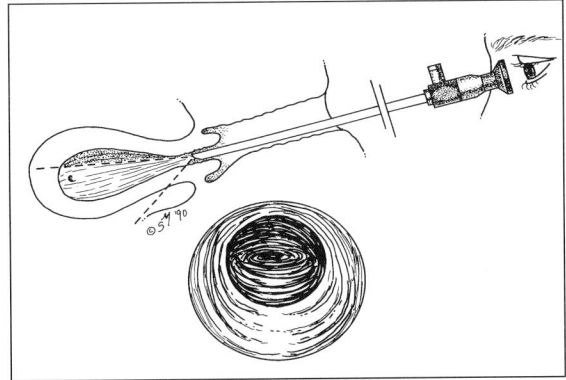

Figure 3.9 Visualization of the uterine cavity with a foreoblique lens: With the light cord facing downwards (left), the anterior wall is better visualized; when the light cord faces upwards (right), the posterior wall is better seen

Selected bibliography

Baggish MS. Distending media for panoramic hysteroscopy. In Baggish MS, Barbot J, Valle RF, eds. *Diagnostic and Operative Hysteroscopy. A Text and Atlas*. Chicago, London, Boca Raton: Year Book Medical Publishers, 1989:89–93

Edstrom K, Fernstrom I. The diagnostic possibilities of a modified hysteroscopic technique. *Acta Obstet Gynecol Scand* 1970;45:327

Lavy G, Diamond MP, Shapiro B, DeCherney AH. A new device to facilitate intrauterine instillation of dextran 70 for hysteroscopy. *Obstet Gynecol* 1987;70:955

Lindemann HJ. The use of CO_2 in the uterine cavity for hysteroscopy. *Int J Fertil* 1972;17:221

Neuwirth RS, Levine RV. Evaluation of a method of hysteroscopy with the use of 30% dextran. *Am J Obstet Gynecol* 1972;114:696

Porto R, Gaujoux J. Une nouvelle methode d'hysteroscopie, instrumentation et technique. *J Gynecol Obstet Biol Reprod* 1972;1:691

Quinones-Guerrero R, Alvarado-Duran A, Aznar-Ramos R. Histeroscopia. Una nueva tecnica. *Ginecol Obstet Mex* 1972;32:337

Quinones RG. Hysteroscopy: Choosing distending media. *Int J Fertil* 1984;29:129

Shirk GJ, Kaigh J. The use of low-viscosity fluids for hysteroscopy. *J Am Assoc Gynecol Laparosc* 1994;2:11

Valle RF, Sciarra JJ. Present status of hysteroscopy in gynecologic practice. *Fertil Steril* 1979;32:619

Valle RF. Hysteroscopy for gynecologic diagnosis. *Clin Obstet Gynecol* 1983;26:253

Valle RF. Hysteroscopy. In Wynn RH, ed. *Obstetrics and Gynecology Annual*. New York: Appleton-Century-Crofts, 1978:245–83

4 Indications and contraindications of hysteroscopy

Before performing any surgical procedure, there must be a specific indication and the benefits obtained by the operation should greatly outweigh the potential risks. The appropriate technique and instrumentation should be established and defined, and there should be no contraindications to the procedure.

The potential applications of hysteroscopy were realized at its inception about a century ago, and its true value has been established by clinical trials which have confirmed the benefits and utility of hysteroscopy in clinical practice. At present, the main indication of its use is to evaluate abnormal uterine bleeding. Furthermore, pathological lesions such as polyps, submucous leiomyomas or focal areas of endometrium suggestive of hyperplasia or carcinoma can be identified, and their location, extension and particular topography assessed to allow determination of the need for selected biopsies or direct treatment (Table 4.1).

Abnormal uterine bleeding

Abnormal uterine bleeding is the main indication for hysteroscopy, particularly in premenopausal women with persistent abnormal bleeding, and bleeding in peri- and postmenopausal patients (Table 4.2). Direct visualization of the uterine cavity increases the accuracy of diagnoses of suspected intrauterine pathology by offering the opportunity to obtain selected biopsies of abnormal or suspicious areas of endome-trium. Although suction aspiration of the endometrium is used routinely in the evaluation of patients with abnormal uterine bleeding, the accuracy and completeness of this evaluation may be limited in the presence of submucous leiomyomas or endometrial polyps and focal areas of endometrium, particularly at the uterotubal junctions.

Table 4.1 Diagnostic applications of hysteroscopy

Exploration of endocervical canal
Suspected endometrial polyps
Suspected submucous leiomyomas
Misplaced foreign bodies
Uterine anomalies
Intrauterine adhesions
Evaluation of endometrial lining
Evaluation of uterotubal junctions
Focal pathologically suspect lesions (endometrial carcinoma and precursors), location, extent

Table 4.2 Indications for hysteroscopy

Evaluate unexplained abnormal uterine bleeding in pre- or postmenopausal patients
Diagnose and / or transcervically remove submucous leiomyomas or polyps
Locate and retrieve 'lost' intrauterine devices and other foreign bodies
Evaluate infertile patients who have abnormal hysterosalpingograms
Diagnose and / or surgically treat intrauterine adhesions
Diagnose and / or surgically treat uterine septa
Explore endocervical canal and uterine cavity in cases of repeated spontaneous abortions
Evaluate failed first-trimester elective abortion
Ablate endometrium in intractable menorrhagia
Cannulate Fallopian tubes

Table 4.3 Hysteroscopic confirmation of hysterographic abnormal findings

Author	Patients with abnormal hysterograms (n)	Confirmed by hysteroscopy (%)
Edstrom & Fernstrom	30	53.3
Englund et al.	21	50.0
Gribb	14	43.0
Levine & Neuwirth	11	50.0
Norment	50	60.0
Porto & Serment	76	58.0
Sugimoto & Nishimura	206	65.0
Taylor & Cumming	68*	55.5
Valle	63	68.3
Varangot et al.+	71	55.0

*Normal hysterograms, only 30 confirmed;
+Contact hysteroscopy

(From Valle & Sciarra, 1979)

Direct visualization of the uterine cavity enhances evaluation of topographical and architectural distortions, allowing visual exploration of the entire uterine cavity.

Hysteroscopy permits targeted biopsies to be taken of abnormal or suspicious areas of endometrium. Because visualization alone cannot adequately distinguish between benign and malignant or premalignant endometrial lesions, biopsies of these lesions are particularly important. In young adolescent patients complaining of abnormal uterine bleeding, the diagnosis can easily be obtained with a clinical history and selected laboratory evaluations to rule out coagulopathies; in adults and particularly those who are peri- or postmenopausal, however, endometrial biopsies are mandatory.

Infertility

Although hysteroscopy is not used routinely to evaluate infertility, it is the best method for confirming or rectifying an abnormal hysterosalpingogram. The latter method of evaluation has a significant rate of false-positives due to transient distortion of the uterine cavity due to blood, mucus, debris and / or air bubbles. Confirmation of an abnormal hysterosalpingogram by subsequent hysteroscopy has varied from 43–68% in comparative studies (Table 4.3).

The abnormal hysterogram is the main indication for hysteroscopy in infertile patients. Hysteroscopy and hysterosalpingography do not exclude each other, but rather are complementary (Table 4.4). The hysterosalpingogram is the basic screening method for evaluating the uterine cavity and Fallopian tubes in the infertile patient. The method is relatively simple and inexpensive, and provides valuable information. When an abnormal hysterosalpingogram is obtained, it is important not only to confirm, but also to determine accurately, the abnormality and plan for treatment. Although, occasionally, hysteroscopy may detect minor abnormalities in a patient with a normal hysterogram, these findings usually are of minor or no clinical significance except when the endometrium is evaluated in patients with abnormal uterine bleeding.

Suspected endometrial polyps and submucous leiomyomas

Hysteroscopy is the best method for diagnosing or confirming endometrial polyps or submucous leiomyomas. Endometrial polyps are due to proliferation and hypertrophy of

Table 4.4 Comparison of hysteroscopy and hysterosalpingography

Hysteroscopy	Hysterosalpingography
Direct visualization of uterine cavity	Indirect visualization (uses contrast-medium shadow)
Diagnosis and specification of intrauterine lesions	Recognition and presumptive diagnosis of intrauterine lesions
Possibility of targeted biopsy and surgical therapy	No possibility of targeted biopsy and surgical therapy
Precise localization of abnormalities (polyps, leiomyomas, malformations, adhesions, carcinoma and precursors)	Localization of abnormalities is less precise
Direct access to tubal lumen (biochemical or biophysical studies, selective chromopertubation)	No direct access (indirect study; possible spasm)
No evaluation of Fallopian tubes possible	Evaluation of tubal lumen, patency, epithelial folds and abnormalities
Requires special instrumentation and experience, and is more costly	Simple instrumentation, easy to perform and less expensive

the basal layer of endometrium. On visualization, the polyp surface shows virtually no vascularization (Figure 4.1) as most vascularization is central, branching peripherally from a central core. The polyps are smooth and soft, and indent easily on contact. Submucous leiomyomas are benign solid tumors composed of muscular fibers and fibrotic connective tissue; in general, except when they have a necrotic surface, they show a peculiar superficial vascularization that is visible through atrophied endometrium (Figure 4.2) which can easily be traced to the base of the myoma. When these superficial vessels are injured, they bleed profusely as they lack a hemostatic mechanism. They feel hard to the touch and cannot be indented easily with probes and forceps. Both types of

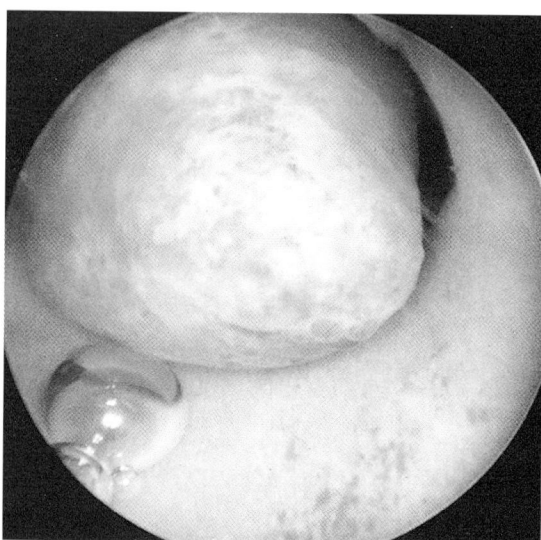

Figure 4.1 Hysteroscopic view of an endometrial polyp

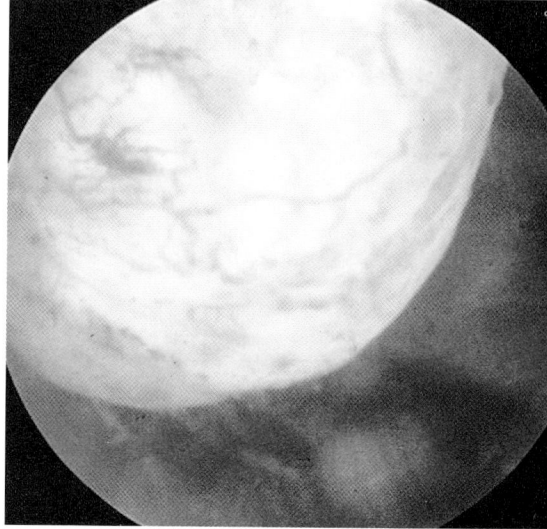

Figure 4.2 Submucous leiomyoma with characteristic peripheral vascularization seen through an atrophic endometrium

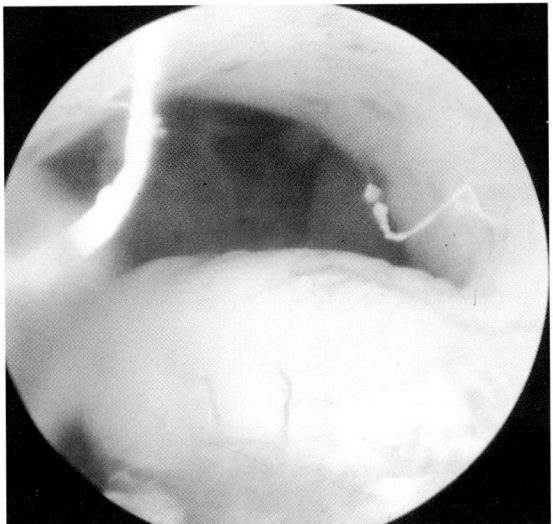

Figure 4.3 This sessile submucous leiomyoma was located in the left lower portion of the uterine cavity

lesions may be sessile or pedunculated (Figure 4.3) and located at different levels of endometrium. Because these lesions distort the symmetry of the uterine cavity, they are easily diagnosed on panoramic visualization of the uterine cavity with a hysteroscope.

Suspected intrauterine adhesions

Scars resulting from trauma in the postpartum or postabortal period may result in menstrual abnormalities such as hypomenorrhea and amenorrhea, depending on the extent of uterine cavity occlusion. The diagnosis is usually suspected from the patient's history and confirmed by hysterosalpingography. To outline the precise distortion of the uterine cavity and permit direct treatment, intrauterine visualization is required. With hysteroscopy, the uterine cavity can be evaluated and its symmetry reestablished on selective division of the adhesions.

To determine the prognosis in the treatment of intrauterine adhesions, it is important to classify the extent of uterine cavity occlusion (Figure 4.4) and the types of adhesions present. Using hysterosalpingography and hysteroscopy, three types of intrauterine adhesions may be defined: mild adhesions are filmy (endometrial) adhesions which produce partial or complete uterine cavity

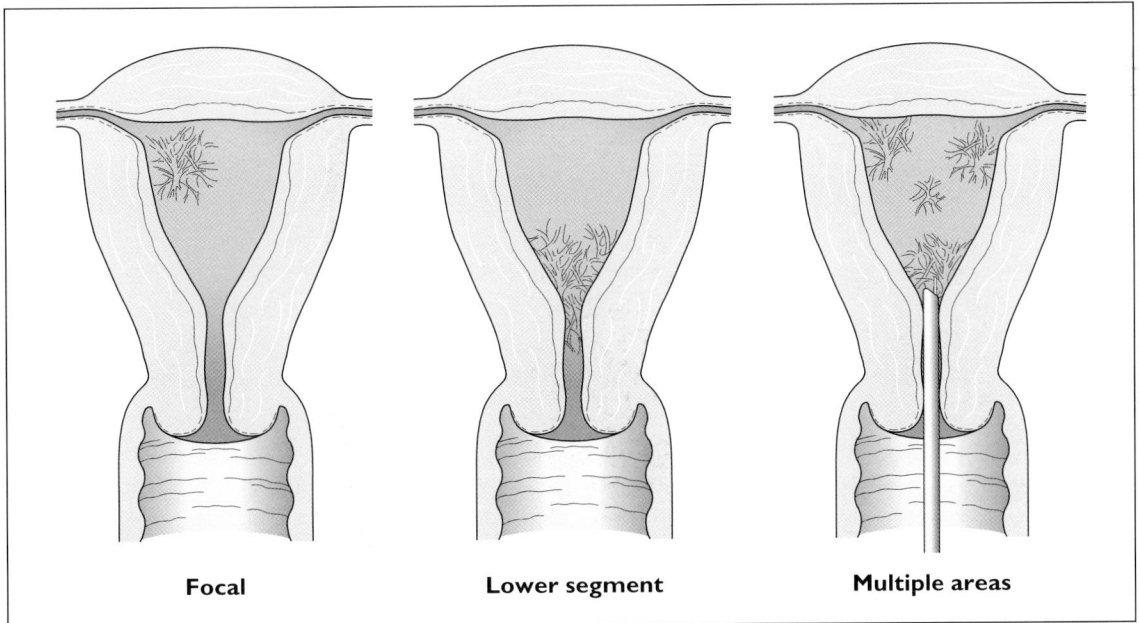

| Focal | Lower segment | Multiple areas |

Figure 4.4 Various presentations of intrauterine adhesions

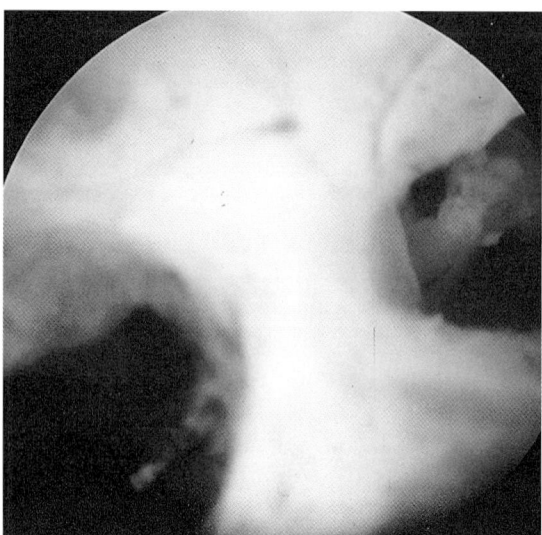

Figure 4.5 This thick adhesion extends from one uterine wall to the other, thereby causing distortion of the uterine cavity

occlusion; moderate adhesions are fibromuscular adhesions that are characteristically thick and covered with endometrium that may bleed upon division, and can partially or totally occlude the uterine cavity (Figure 4.5); severe adhesions are composed of connective tissue only with no endometrial lining, are unlikely to bleed upon division and may partially or totally occlude the uterine cavity. The more fibrotic the adhesions, the worse the prognosis and, thus, the thinner and more recent the adhesions, the better the prognosis.

Evaluation and confirmation of uterine anomalies

Uterine septa

Approximately 25% of women with a septate uterus experience reproductive wastage. The classical clinical picture is that of repeated early mid-trimester abortions with signs of labor and bleeding. By tradition, when women with repetitive abortions due to

uterine septation require treatment, abdominal metroplasty either by excision of the septum through a wedge uterine excision (Jones) or by incision of the septum without excision of tissue (Tompkins) has been performed. Both operations require laparotomy and hysterotomy, with their concomitant inconvenience, hospitalization and prolonged recovery.

Uterine septa may vary in length, be either partial or complete, or involve the cervix as well. Septal thickness varies from thin to thick and wide. Furthermore, when uterine septa are present, other uterine pathology, such as polyps, myomas or intrauterine adhesions, may be encountered.

Because uterine septa are often poorly vascularized, hysteroscopy is used to divide the septum transcervically under direct vision; the procedure was previously attempted blind by a few practitioners, but abandoned due to the difficulties involved.

Tubal ostia

The first 2–3 mm into the tubal ostia can be evaluated by hysteroscopy. Although partial tubal cannulation was first performed in the late 1960s, the technique was not refined until the early 1970s, with experience gained from tubal sterilization. Hysteroscopic evaluation of the intramural Fallopian tubes provides an opportunity to treat polyps and adhesions obstructing or distorting the tubal ostia. Because the first 2–3 mm of the Fallopian tube is not markedly convoluted, direct ostial cannulation, performed since the early 1970s, allows the selective assessment of tubal patency.

Several pathological conditions may be diagnosed at the tubal openings. These include polyps occluding the tubes, adhesions and rigid or sclerotic tubal ostia that do not respond well to stimuli and produce physiological spasms that may inhibit opening and closing with intrauterine pressure. The first 2–3 mm of tubal epithelium can also be visualized and evaluated by hysteroscopy (Figures 4.6–4.8).

Other clinical applications

Hysteroscopy is of value in exploring the cervical canal in patients who have had repeated abortions. Visual appraisal of the cervical canal during hysteroscopic examination reveals that, in many of these patients, there is a loss of the anatomical relationship between the corpus and the cervix, and disappearance of the sphincter-like action of the internal cervical os. Uterine anomalies can also be detected.

Adenomyosis

Adenomyosis is difficult to diagnose consistently with hysteroscopy and is only occasionally suspected if small sinuses are observed, particularly in the fundal region. The condition is also difficult to diagnose

by biopsy taken through the hysteroscope or even with the resectoscope, as only superficial myometrial tissue can thus be obtained. The best method available for the diagnosis of adenomyosis is by magnetic resonance imaging (MRI), particularly if the patient reports abnormal uterine bleed-

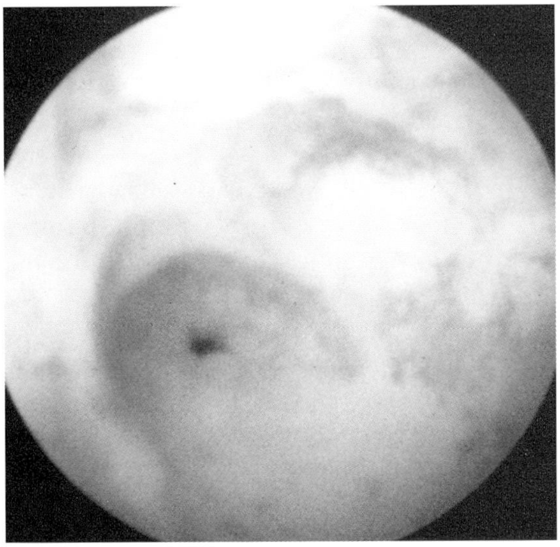

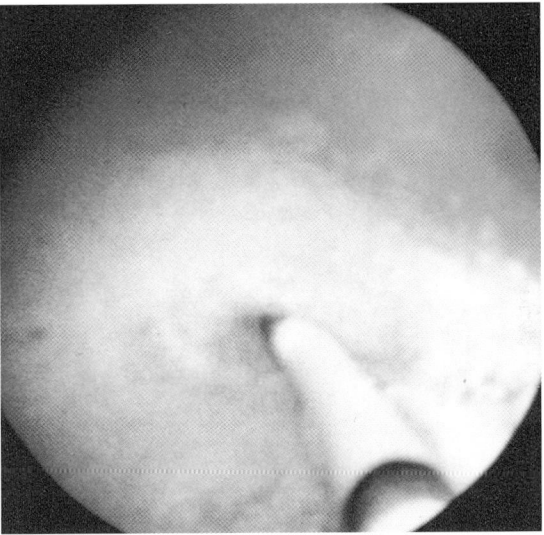

Figure 4.7 Hysteroscopic cannulation of the tubal ostium

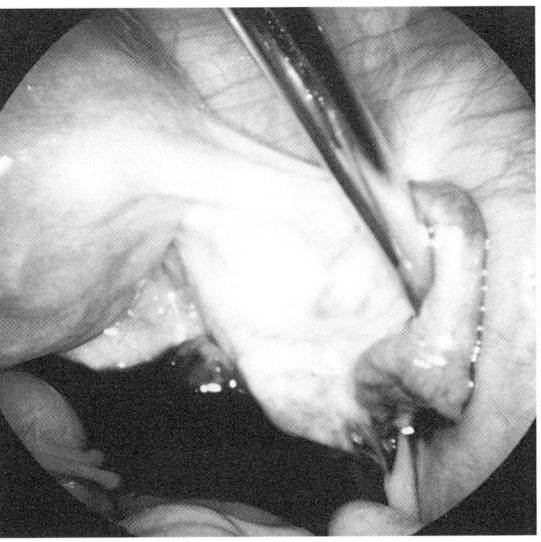

Figure 4.8 Chromopertubation shows tubal patency at laparoscopy after cannulation

Figure 4.6 Hysteroscopic view of the uterotubal junction

ing and cyclical pain, although vaginal ultrasound can measure myometrial thickness.

Tubaloscopy

Tubaloscopy has been attempted since the late 1960s, using the hysteroscope as the conduit for miniendoscopes or falloposcopes; manufacturers are now developing new miniendoscopes that improve the field of view and resolution, and also offer the capability of washing and introducing fluids while maintaining a diameter of less than 1mm. The miniendoscope is still being investigated and cannot be routinely used for transcervical evaluation of the Fallopian tubes.

Although the ability to examine the tubal lumen from the uterine side has developed with the introduction of hysteroscopy, achieving a clear and distinct view of the tubal lumen has been difficult due to the limitations of technology. It is possible to pass small catheters into the tubal lumen, but the view obtained with the microendoscopes is poor with low resolution. Such small-diameter endoscopes cannot provide adequate flushing and distention of the tube to permit the endoscope to be advanced from the uterus.

The best evaluation is obtained during withdrawal of the endoscope. Endoscopy of the ampulla and distal end of the tube is best performed with rigid endoscopes 3 mm in diameter introduced from the abdominal side. This permits excellent distention and visualization, thereby allowing the recognition and evaluation of these anatomical structures.

Tubal endoscopy from the uterus remains a research tool waiting for technology to provide the appropriate endoscopes to allow clear and distinct evaluation of the structures and topography of the intramural and isthmic tubal lumen.

Embryoscopy

Although it is possible to introduce mini-endoscopes transcervically to observe the early embryo, the optical resolution has not been satisfactory. Rigid miniendoscopes can now be introduced transabdominally and transuterine to observe the embryo *in situ* with better resolution. As the technology advances, the possibility of a practical transcervical method for embryoscopy remains on the horizon. As miniendoscopes become accepted for intrauterine visualization, the transfer of gametes, zygotes or embryos under visual control may become a reality.

The fundamental elements needed to perform hysteroscopy on the embryo include an appropriate hysteroscope, a uterine-distending medium, an illumination source and ancillary instrumentation.

When an early first-trimester pregnancy termination fails and histological examination of the products of conception does not demonstrate chorionic villi, an ectopic pregnancy should be suspected, particularly if the pregnancy test is persistently positive. When laparoscopy fails to demonstrate tubal pathology and / or lesions of the ovary or peritoneal layer consistent with an ectopic pregnancy, hysteroscopy may be of value. The reason may be early gestation in an anomalous uterus, such as a septate uterus with an early pregnancy at a site that was not curetted. Hysteroscopy can guide selective suction aspiration for termination of the missed pregnancy.

Although the indications of hysteroscopy are well established, other potential hysteroscopic diagnostic applications remain under investigation. Changes in the topography of the endometrium during the menstrual cycle have been evaluated by correlation of the superficial vascularization patterns and changes in the endometrial glandular openings as the cycle progresses with the degree of endometrial maturation. Miniaturization of endoscopes permits less traumatic access for tubal cannulation of the Fallopian tubes, and may open the door to better evaluation of the Fallopian tubes and to applications for new reproductive technologies. The hysteroscope remains an attractive tool for eventual achievement of tubal sterilization.

In summary, the most common indications for hysteroscopy are: evaluation of abnormal, persistent or recurrent uterine bleeding; evaluation of an abnormal hysterogram; surgical treatment of intrauterine adhesions; division of uterine septa; removal of submucous leiomyomas; location and removal of misplaced intrauterine devices; tubal cannulation in patients with tubal cornual occlusions; and endometrial ablation (destruction).

Contraindications of hysteroscopy

Some contraindications are absolute in that hysteroscopy should never be performed when these contraindications are present. Others are relative, and indicate that the technique must be modified and the patients individually selected for this approach.

Absolute contraindications are pelvic inflammatory disease and profuse uterine bleeding. Pelvic inflammatory disease is an absolute contraindication because of the potential of spreading infection, through either the bloodstream or lymphatic routes systemically, or Fallopian tubes into the peritoneal cavity. Infection must be ruled out in patients presenting with symptoms or a history of recent pelvic infection by appropriate cervical cultures before hysteroscopy to prevent exacerbation of an existing infection, and by applying meticulous attention to technique to avoid introduction of new infection to the endometrial cavity.

Profuse uterine bleeding can make hysteroscopy cumbersome regardless of the distending medium used. If bleeding is not excessive, proper evacuation and washing of the endometrial cavity prior to uterine distention may permit adequate, albeit temporary, visualization.

Relative contraindications are desired pregnancy, cervical malignancy, menstruation, known adenocarcinoma of the endometrium, cervical stenosis, recent uterine perforation and operator inexperience.

Pregnancy

Hysteroscopy is contraindicated during pregnancy, as the possibility of infection or interruption of a wanted pregnancy far outweighs the value of intrauterine observation. Nonetheless, under special circumstances such as removal of misplaced intrauterine devices in early pregnancy, visualization may be performed in selected patients, with the technique modified to decrease the chances of interrupting the pregnancy. It is important to weigh the benefits derived from hysteroscopy during early pregnancy against the potential of damaging or interrupting the pregnancy.

Cervical malignancy

In the presence of known cervical malignancy, manipulation of the area should be avoided to prevent possible spread. Patients with known carcinoma of the cervix should not be subjected to hysteroscopy particularly because the information derived may not contribute to the plan of treatment. Nonetheless, under meticulous and controlled protocols, the endocervical canal can be evaluated with a small-caliber endoscope to assess the extent of an adenocarcinoma of the cervix. This evaluation should be carried out in conjunction with a gynecological oncologist to establish a proper plan of therapy.

Menstruation

Hysteroscopy should not be performed during menstruation to avoid potential risks of infection from necrotic tissue; menstrual blood could potentially be pushed through the Fallopian tubes into the peritoneal cavity by distention. However, if necessary, hysteroscopy could be performed with a continuous-flow hysteroscope that permits continuous washing of blood and debris under low intrauterine pressures to avoid transtubal reflux. Hysteroscopy is best performed following the completion of menstruation.

Adenocarcinoma of endometrium

Hysteroscopy is used in the evaluation of patients with abnormal uterine bleeding. Occasionally, abnormal focal areas of endometrium are found and confirmed to be carcinoma. However, in a patient with known carcinoma of endometrium, the use of hysteroscopy should be cautiously undertaken particularly because, at that stage, a carcinoma is likely to be extensive and adding hysteroscopy may not change the plan of treatment. If it is necessary to determine involvement of the cervix, hysteroscopy may be used in collaboration with a gynecological oncologist to evaluate the extent of the adenocarcinoma and confirm involvement of the cervical canal.

Cervical stenosis

When the endocervical canal cannot be dilated adequately to introduce the endo-scope, hysteroscopy cannot be performed. With the use of small-caliber endoscopes, the procedure may be facilitated, but if the endoscope, despite a small caliber, cannot be passed through the cervical canal under direct vision, the procedure cannot be performed safely.

Recent uterine perforation

If the uterus cannot be distended adequately due to a uterine wall defect, hysteroscopy becomes cumbersome. The patient should be allowed to heal and the examination performed at a later time. Nonetheless, perforation with a small-caliber endoscope may not preclude uterine distention if appropriate precautions are taken. When a small perforation has occurred, hysteroscopy may be attempted with a continuous-flow system to permit continuous lavage. If this does not permit uterine distention, then laparoscopy may help in occluding the small perforation from the abdominal side while hysteroscopy is being performed.

Operator inexperience

Attempting hysteroscopy without proper training and supervision may convert a simple technique into a potential source of complications. Of all the contraindications, that of greatest concern is cervical or uterine infection without obvious clinical symptoms. Fortunately, active infection following hysteroscopic examination is rare. Nonetheless, strict adherence to a combination of proper indications, absence of contraindications, meticulous technique and an experienced surgeon pave the way for a procedure performed without serious complications or sequelae.

Selected bibliography

Ahumada JC, Gandolfo-Herrera R. Histeroscopia. *Rev Med Lat Am* 1935;21:265

Bordt J, Belkien L, Vancaillie, *et al.* Ergebnisse diagnostischer hysteroskopien in einem IVF/ET-Programm. *Gerburts Frauenheilk* 1984; 44:813

Ghilardini G, Gualerzi C, Fachi F, *et al.* Chorionoscopy and chorionic villi sampling. *Acta Eur Fertil* 1986;17:491

van Herendael B, Stevens M, Flakiewicz-Kula A, Hansch C. Dating of the endometrium by microhysteroscopy. *Gynecol Obstet Invest* 1987;24:11

Kerin J, Dayhovsky L, Segalowitz J, *et al.* Falloposcopy: A microendoscopic technique for visual exploration of the human fallopian tube from the uterotubal ostium to the fimbria using a transvaginal approach. *Fertil Steril* 1990;54:390

Mencaglia L, Ricci G, Perino A, *et al.* Hysteroscopic chorionic villi sampling: A new approach. *Acta Eur Fertil* 1986;17:495

Menken FC. Endoscopic observations of endocrine processes and hormonal changes. In Ruiz-Albretch F, Ramirez-Sanchez J, Willowitzer H, eds. *Simposio sobre Esteroides Sexuales.* Berlin: Saladruck, 1969:276

Norment WB. Hysteroscope in diagnosis of pathological conditions of uterine canal. *J Am Med Assoc* 1952;148:917

Norment WB, Sikes CH, Berry FX, Bird I. Hysteroscopy. *Surg Clin North Am* 1957; 37:1377

Novy MJ, Thurmond AS, Patton P, *et al.* Diagnosis of cornual obstructions by transcervical fallopian tube cannulation. *Fertil Steril* 1988; 50:434

Pantaleoni DC. An endoscopic examination of the cavity of the womb. *Med Press Circ (Lond)* 1969;8:26

Quinones-Guerrero R, Alvarado-Duran, Aznar-Ramos R. Tubal catheterization: Applications of a new technique. *Am J Obstet Gynecol* 1972;114:674

Quinones-Guerrero R, Aznar-Ramos R, Alvarado-Duran A. Tubal electrocauterization under hysteroscopic control. *Contraception* 1973;7:195

Sciarra JJ, Butler JC, Speidel JJ, eds. *Hysteroscopic Sterilization.* New York: Intercontinental Medical Book Corporation, 1974

Sciarra JJ, Valle RF. Hysteroscopy. A clinical experience with 320 patients. *Am J Obstet Gynecol* 1977;127:340

Snowden EU, Jarret JC, Dawood MY. Comparison of diagnostic accuracy of laparoscopy, hysteroscopy, and hysterosalpingography in evaluation of female infertility. *Fertil Steril* 1984;41:709

Valle RF, Sciarra JJ. Current status of hysteroscopy in gynecologic practice. *Fertil Steril* 1979;32: 619

Valle RF. Hysteroscopic evaluation of patients with abnormal uterine bleeding. *Surg Gynecol Obstet* 1981;153:521

Valle RF. Hysteroscopy in the evaluation of female infertility. *Am J Obstet Gynecol* 1980;137:425

Valle RF, Sabbagha RS. Management of first trimester pregnancy termination failures. *Obstet Gynecol* 1989;73:201

Valle RF. Future growth and development of hysteroscopy. In DeCherney AH, ed. *Hysteroscopy*. Philadelphia, PA: WB Saunders, 1988:111–26

Valle RF. Indications for hysteroscopy. In Siegler AM, Lindemann HJ, eds. *Hysteroscopy: Principles and Practice*. Philadelphia, PA: JB Lippincott, 1984:21–4

Valle RF. Hysteroscopy for gynecologic diagnosis. In Baggish MS, ed. *Gynecologic Endoscopy and Instrumentation. Clinical Obstetrics and Gynecology*. Hagerstown, MD: Harper & Row, 1983:253–76

5 Possible complications of hysteroscopy

Because hysteroscopy is a surgical technique requiring manipulation of the cervix and uterus, and dissection and removal of intrauterine pathological lesions, it has the potential for complications. These complications may be related to the procedure itself, distending medium, specific surgical procedures performed, additional techniques or instrumentation that may be required or to the anesthesia.

Procedural complications

Complications related to the procedure itself are similar to those that occur during intrauterine manipulations such as curettage. These include laceration of the cervix by a tenaculum, uterine perforation and infection. Cervical laceration from the tenaculum can occur when excessive manipulation is performed by traction, but can easily be corrected by suturing the defect and prevented by gentle manipulation. While minor lacerations can occur while placing the tenaculum in the cervix, bleeding can only occur if the uterine walls are damaged or a vascular tumor is disturbed. Uterine perforation can occur either during blind uterine sounding before hysteroscopy or when the hysteroscope is advanced blindly and forcibly into the uterine cavity. This type of perforation can be prevented by not advancing the endoscope unless a panoramic view is accomplished by adequate uterine distention. The use of a uterine sound is seldom required as the endoscope is guided under direct vision.

When these complications occur, the treatment varies according to the size and location of the perforation. Perforation with a uterine sound seldom requires treatment (Figures 5.1–5.3). If a uterine perforation occurs, the procedures of hysteroscopy should be avoided altogether and the patient observed for possible decompensation. When uterine perforation is due to a large operative hysteroscope, further evaluation may be necessary, including laparoscopy to assess persistent bleeding and to accomplish hemostasis. During operative procedures, should perforation occur with mechanical instrumentation, the treatment usually does not differ from perforations due to the hysteroscope itself. If perforation occurs when additional techniques such as electrosurgery or a laser are used, further evaluation is mandatory to rule out damage to adjacent structures. If laparoscopic evaluation is negative, patients should be followed closely for signs of infection, early intestinal obstruction and / or delayed hemorrhage.

Infection, although possible when an endoscope is introduced into the uterine cavity, is rare when precautions such as disinfection and sterilization of instruments are taken. The appropriate selection, evaluation and preparation of patients for hysteroscopy helps to prevent infection. To avoid contamination of the cervical canal and uterine cavity during the procedure, sterile techniques should be maintained and protocols meticulously followed.

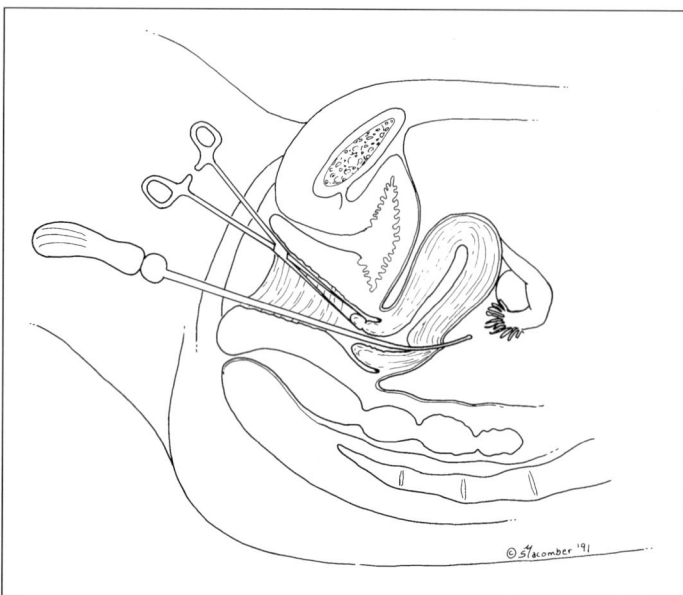

Figure 5.1 Posterior uterine perforation by a uterine sound

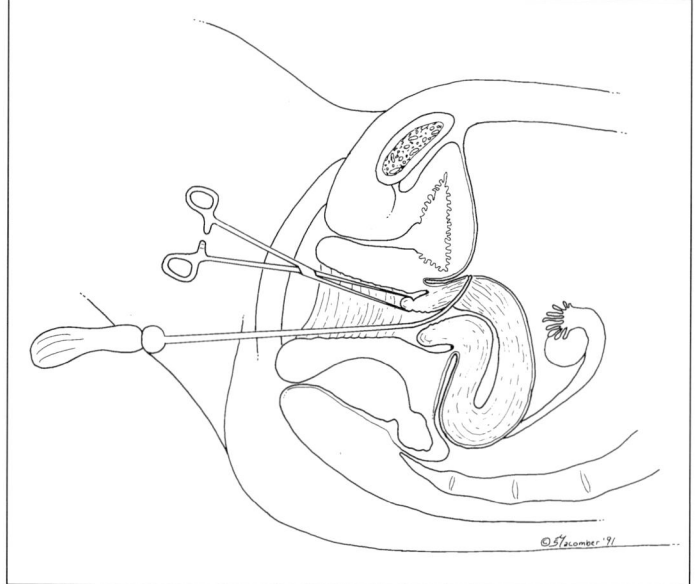

Figure 5.2 Anterior uterine perforation by a uterine sound in a retroverted uterus

Complications with distending media

Complications related to distending media vary according to the medium. When CO_2 gas exceeds the flow rate of 100 mL / min, hypercapnia, arrhythmias, acidosis and even gas emboli may occur. These problems can be avoided by using machines specifically designed for hysteroscopy which electronically calibrate the appropriate flow rate of about 40–60 mL / min and do not permit intrauterine pressures > 100–150 mmHg. Other machines not specifically designed for hysteroscopy, particularly those used for laparoscopy, should never be used to distend the uterus. When low-viscosity fluids are used to distend the uterine cavity during

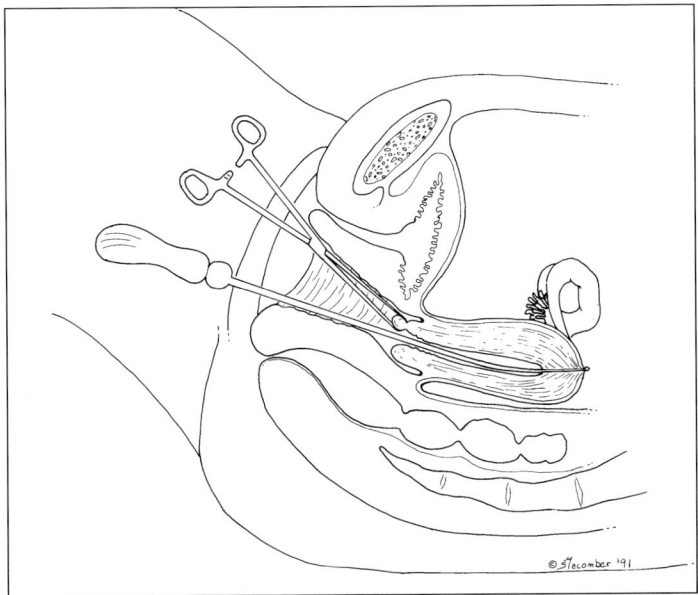

Figure 5.3 Fundal perforation by a uterine sound

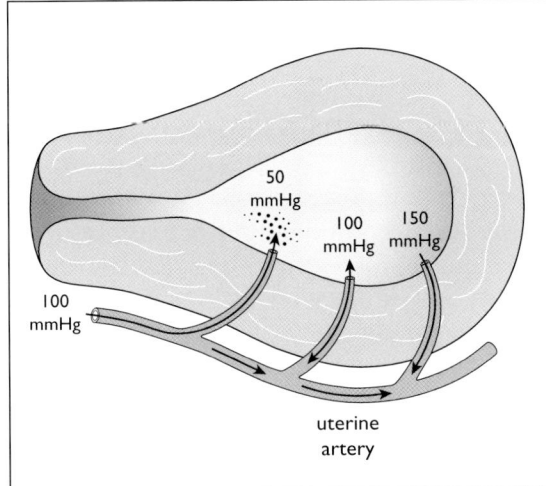

Figure 5.4 Titration of intrauterine pressure against mean arterial pressure

operative hysteroscopy, the most frequent complications are secondary to fluid overload and electrolyte imbalance, particularly if fluids devoid of electrolytes are used. It is important, therefore, to control meticulously the quantity of fluids administered and to measure the quantity of fluids recovered. Furthermore, the intrauterine pressure should be kept below the mean arterial pressure of 100 mmHg (Figure 5.4).

Although there is no specific standard quantity of non-recovered fluids or deficit that is absolutely safe, several parameters alert the endoscopist to early decompensation. When fluids with electrolytes are used, the threshold of toxicity or decompensation may be increased, as significant diuresis may compensate for the fluid overload in the early stages. When prolonged procedures are performed and significant dissections are required, it is important to measure urine output with an indwelling catheter to assure no oliguria or anuria occurs. The anesthesiologist should carefully monitor vital signs such as blood pressure, pulse and pulse oximetry. The circulating nurse should meticulously measure the fluid introduced or injected as well as the fluid recovered to have an accurate periodic account of the deficit.

Fluids containing electrolytes are less likely to cause serious problems. Fluid overload cannot be totally avoided, but precautionary measures such as early diuretic use can be implemented to prevent intravasation of excessive amounts of fluid. Hyponatremia is avoided and the threshold for toxicity increased as the patient maintains diuresis.

In general, a deficit of no more than 1000–1500 mL of fluid containing electrolytes should be permitted. This amount, although conservative, will certainly prevent major fluid overload. If the quantity of non-recovered fluid detected is excessive, particularly with signs of decompensation in the vital signs or urine output, the operation should be stopped and diuretics administered under close monitoring.

When fluids devoid of electrolytes are used, precautions in addition to monitoring should be undertaken. Should a deficit of 700–800 mL occur, the operation should be stopped and a stat serum sodium determined. If no lowering of the serum sodium has occurred, the operation may proceed providing that only a short time is required to complete the procedure. However, if the serum sodium is lower than normal and the required operation is prolonged, the procedure should be aborted and completed at another time. Further decompensation in the serum sodium with deficits > 1000 mL should be immediately and appropriately corrected. The use of diuretics under these circumstances should be undertaken with caution and meticulous monitoring of serum electrolytes.

When using dextran 70 32% for operative procedures, it is important to measure the amount of dextran infused and the amount recovered to prevent more than 300 mL being absorbed by the patient. When greater quantities are absorbed by intravasation of the dextran under pressure, a non-cardiogenic pulmonary edema may occur, perhaps due to the osmotic effect of the dextran shifting fluids to the intravascular system. Additionally, because of the effect of dextran on coagulation factors, a coagulopathy similar to disseminated intravascular coagulation may ensue, with decreasing platelets, a prolonged partial thromboplastin time and low fibrinogen. This condition should be recognized and immediately treated with respiratory support measures, cautious use of diuretics and plasmapheresis for degradation of the large molecules of dextran; if coagulopathy ensues, appropriate therapy should be given. Allergic reactions to dextran, although unusual, may occur and require appropriate management. In such cases, the operation should be immediately discontinued, and the patient provided with therapeutic support of circulatory and respiratory systems.

If a procedure is expected to be prolonged, monitoring is mandatory. If the procedure cannot be completed with a limited amount of dextran, other alternatives should be instituted, including low-viscosity fluids with or without electrolytes, depending on the procedure and the type of energy used.

Complications of anesthesia

Complications may be related to the anesthetic used. Local anesthetics may on occasions cause allergic reactions, but the most common complications are due to intravasation. Therefore, the type of anesthetic used, whether an ester or amide, should be known. The toxicity of these anesthetics should be kept in mind and, when problems of intravasation occur, they should be appropriately handled. Usually, intravenous diazepam corrects the problem. Anesthetics of the ester type, such as chloroprocaine (Nesacaine®) and mercaine, have a low toxicity and, when intravasation occurs, their rapid degradation by the plasma pseudocholinesterase helps in their elimination. Because only a small amount is generally required for paracervical block, 3–4 mL in each uterosacral ligament, toxicity is markedly decreased.

Problems related to general anesthesia and regional anesthetics are the responsibility of the anesthesiologist.

Complications of lasers in operative hysteroscopy

When using fiberoptic lasers, it is important to use either the bare fiber, or sculpted or extruded fibers, and to avoid coaxial fibers, particularly those fitted with sapphire tips as they require continuous cooling by gases or fluids. Indeed, the latter lasers should never be used in the uterus to avoid massive intravasation of gas or air developing into a fatal gas embolus. When using these fine fiberoptic lasers to operate in the uterus, perforation of the uterine wall can occur if the laser is pressed too quickly into the uterine wall. Perforation can be avoided by operating at all times under direct view with great caution and attention to detail. If perforation occurs while the laser is activated, injury to other organs is possible. Because of the reflective nature of these lasers and their attraction to pigments, the operator and assistants should protect their eyes with special goggles or filters to avoid retinal injuries.

Complications of electrosurgery

Electrosurgery may cause complications. Because a monopolar current is used, the patient should be properly grounded with an appropriate ground plate serving as a return electrode. Only insulated electrodes and probes should be used; the machines delivering this type of energy should be properly calibrated and have a display of the selected waveform and watt power. Electrosurgery should never be activated without a precise and complete view of the area to be treated, and only fluids devoid of electrolytes should be used to distend the uterine cavity.

Complications from other procedures

Complications resulting from hysteroscopy vary according to the type of procedure performed. The most common complications related to hysteroscopic surgery are bleeding and uterine perforation. These can occur during division of uterine septa or intrauterine adhesions, treatment of myomas, endometrial ablation and tubal cannulation. Because some of these procedures require more time than others, it is important to monitor the fluids used during these procedures to prevent excessive absorption by the patient and fluid overload. Perforation of the uterus may also predispose the patient to injuries to other organs in the pelvic cavity. Therefore, when difficult procedures are performed, particularly if symmetry of the uterine cavity is markedly distorted, concomitant laparoscopy is a helpful adjunct to prevent additional injuries to adjacent organs should perforation occur. While infection with this type of hysteroscopic procedure is uncommon, prophylactic antibiotics are selectively used in some patients, particularly those hoping to preserve fertility by treatment of septa, adhesions and tubal cannulation.

Ideally, no complications should follow any procedure or, when they occur, they should be justified by the need for and benefits derived from the procedure to respect the dictum of *primum non nocere*. Close attention to technique, selection of patients and appropriate performance of each procedure is of utmost importance.

Selected bibliography

Arieff AI, Ayres JC. Endometrial ablation complicated by fatal hyponatremic encephalopathy. *J Am Med Assoc* 1993;270:1230

Baggish MS, Brill AF, Rosenzweig B, *et al.* Fatal acute glycine and sorbitol toxicity during operative hysteroscopy. *J Gynecol Surg* 1993; 9:137

Gallinat A. The effect of carbon dioxide during hysteroscopy. In van der Pas H, van Herendael BJ, van Lith DAF, Keith LG, eds. *Hysteroscopy*. Boston, The Hague, Dordrecht, Lancaster: MTP Press, 1983:19–27

Garry R, Hasham F, Kokri MS, Mooney P. The effect of pressure on fluid absorption during endometrial ablation. *J Gynecol Surg* 1992;8:1

Hulka JF, Peterson HB, Phillips JM, Surrey MW. Operative hysteroscopy. American Association of Gynecologic Laparoscopists 1991 membership survey. *J Reprod Med* 1993; 38:572

Loffer FD. Complications from uterine distention during hysteroscopy. In Corfman RS, Diamond M, DeCherney A, eds. *Complications of Laparoscopy and Hysteroscopy*. Oxford, London, Edinburgh: Blackwell Scientific Publications, 1993:177–86

McLucas B. Hyskon complications in hysteroscopic surgery. *Obstet Gynecol Survey* 1991; 46:196

Nachum Z, Kol S, Adir Y, Melomed Y. Massive air embolism – a possible cause of death after operative hysteroscopy using a 32% dextran 70 pump. *Fertil Steril* 1992;58:836

Peterson HB, Hulka JF, Phillips JM. American Association of Gynecologic Laparoscopists 1988 membership survey on operative hysteroscopy. *J Reprod Med* 1990;25:590

Valle RF. Cervical and uterine complications during insertion of the hysteroscope. In Corfman RS, Diamond M, DeCherney A, eds. *Complications of Laparoscopy and Hysteroscopy*. Oxford, London, Edinburgh: Blackwell Scientific Publications, 1993: 167–76

Witz CA, Silverberg KM, Burns WN, *et al.* Complications associated with the absorption of hysteroscopic fluid media. *Fertil Steril* 1993;60:745

6 Diagnostic hysteroscopy in the office

Office hysteroscopy became practical with the introduction of small-caliber endoscopes (<4 mm in outer diameter) permitting its use in the office setting without the need for cervical dilatation. The small-caliber hysteroscope simplifies examination and allows an easy, safe and expeditious investigation of the uterine cavity. Nonetheless, the small-caliber endoscope has inherent drawbacks. Operative instruments cannot be passed through these small hysteroscopes and only CO_2 gas can be used for uterine distention. However, these small hysteroscopes allow diagnostic hysteroscopy to be performed quickly and simply without the need for anesthesia and / or analgesia.

Thus, the hysteroscope used in an office setting can only serve diagnostic purposes (Figure 6.1). The distending medium is CO_2 gas delivered by a hysterosufflator that electronically maintains the flow rate at a constant 40–50 mL / min and permits an intrauterine pressure of no more than 100–150 mmHg when the Fallopian tubes are open. As the intrauterine pressure increases, the flow rate decreases and *vice versa*. While endoscopes with an outer diameter >4 mm have been developed for use in the office, they are cumbersome; cervical dilatation is often necessary and the patient requires more local anesthetic or sedation. The cervical canal is traumatized, and the uterine cavity

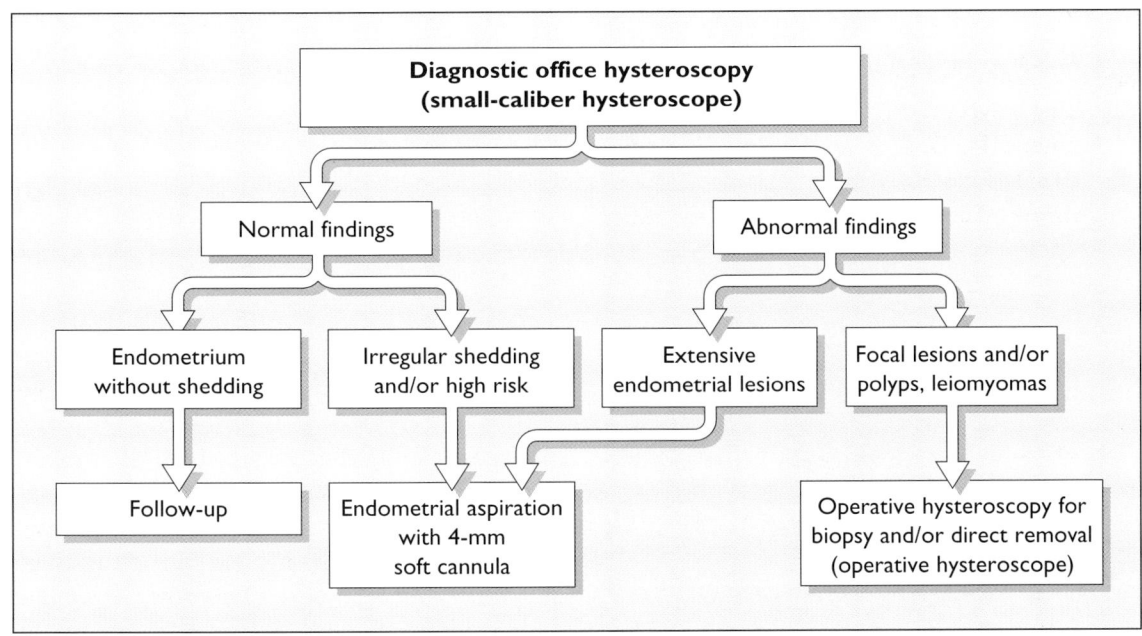

Figure 6.1 Algorithm for hysteroscopic uterine evaluation using diagnostic endoscopes

may contain debris and blood clots that cause the CO_2 gas to bubble inside the cavity, obscuring the view. Whereas endoscopes with diameters > 4 mm may provide a system for washing the cavity with fluids, this method is also cumbersome in the office due to the additional tubing and collection bags for the fluid. Only if the system is simplified and adapted to individual settings can the latter method be an option for office hysteroscopy (Figure 6.2).

The patient selected for hysteroscopy requires a pelvic examination, and disinfection of the vagina and cervix with an antiseptic solution such as povidone iodine

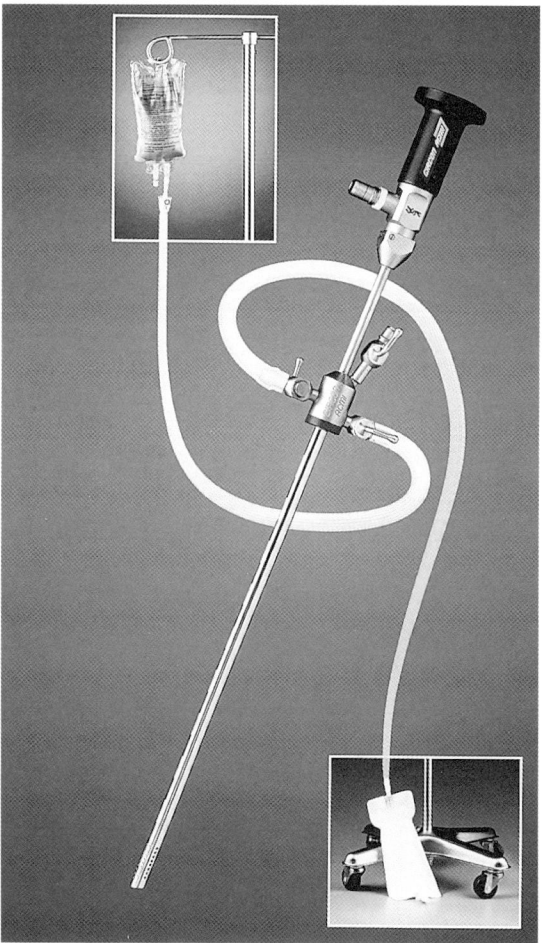

Figure 6.2 Fluid management system simplified for uterine distention in the office

(Betadine®). In general, no systemic sedatives or medications are required as the procedure is practically painless. A paracervical block with 3–4 mL of a local anesthetic, preferably an ester type such as chloroprocaine hydrochloride (Nesacaine 1%), is injected at the base of each uterosacral ligament, close to the cervix and superficially so as to blanch when injected to avoid rapid diffusion (Figure 6.3). A small amount (0.5 mL) at the site where the tenaculum is to be placed is useful (Figure 6.4). Once this is accomplished, a diagnostic hysteroscope with its light source and flowing CO_2 gas is introduced under direct vision to the level of the ectocervix, and the examination begins by slowly and systematically following the small microcavity produced by the CO_2 gas in front of the endoscope. Once the endocervical canal is completely explored (Figure 6.5), the endoscope is advanced across the internal cervical os to allow evaluation of the panoramic view of the uterine cavity, including the uterotubal cornua and tubal ostia. The uterine cavity is reexamined, as is the endocervical canal, during withdrawal of the instrument.

Because these examinations are diagnostic, any pathology found will require either biopsy or hysteroscopic removal. Should therapeutic hysteroscopy be needed, a larger instrument may be required. The decision as to whether this can be performed safely in the office, or in an ambulatory surgical center or operating room suite under local, regional or general anesthesia will depend on the lesion treated. Patients with normal findings at diagnostic hysteroscopy are spared any other manipulation or biopsy. On completion of the hysteroscopic examination, in patients with abnormal uterine bleeding but normal hysteroscopic findings, who nonetheless have abnormal irregular shedding of the endometrial lining, as is usually the case in patients with abnormal

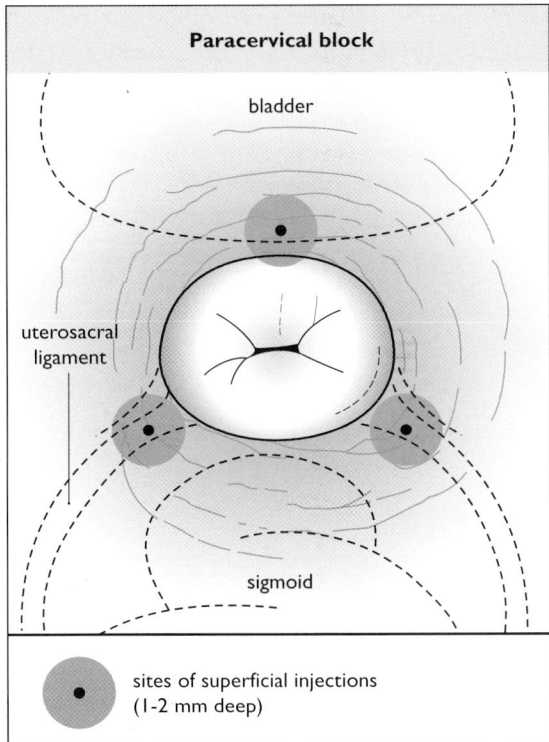

Figure 6.3 Sites of superficial injections (1–2 mm in depth) of anesthetic for a paracervical block

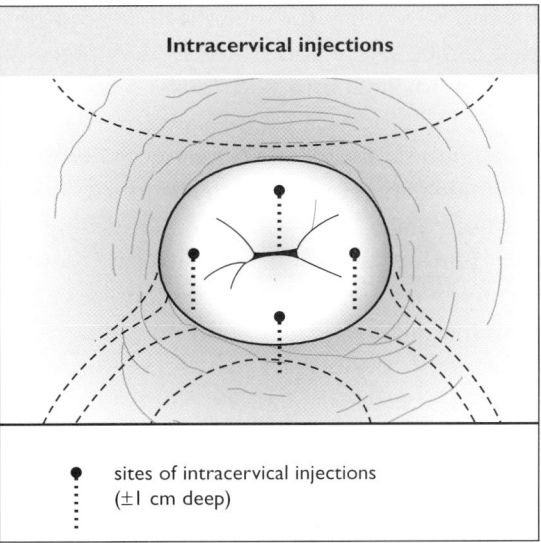

Figure 6.4 Intracervical injections are approximately 1 cm in depth

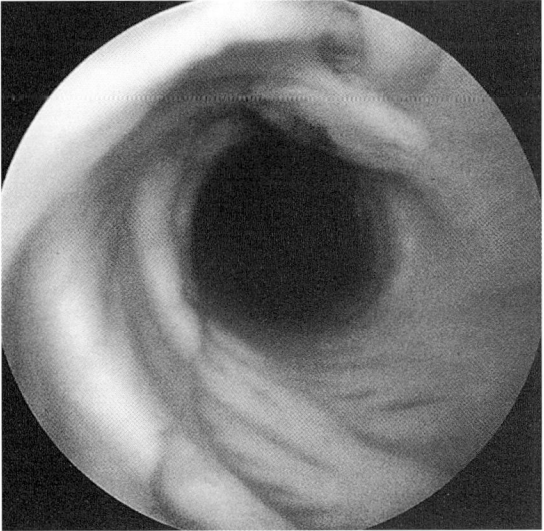

Figure 6.5 Hysteroscopic view of the cervical canal

uterine bleeding, a 4-mm soft plastic cannula is introduced and suction curettage performed for histological evaluation. Because the patient has had a paracervical block, this suction aspiration is usually well tolerated.

Hysteroscopy has been facilitated as a simple office procedure with the use of small-caliber endoscopes. Because of its simplicity and ease of application, hysteroscopy is useful as a screening method for patients with abnormal uterine bleeding and / or questionable hysterograms, and for patients with suspected intrauterine pathology.

Although hysteroscopy can be performed in an office with an operative hysteroscope with a 7-mm outer diameter, the required cervical dilatation and manipulation usually involves additional assistance and attention to detail as well as safety measures in anticipation of such side effects

as bradycardia and / or hypotension. The procedure is similar to that described for office hysteroscopy except that the endocervical canal is gradually dilated to the diameter of a number 7 Hegar (or whichever specific operative hysteroscope is to be used). Despite the feasibility of introducing an operative hysteroscope under paracervical block anesthesia, the operative procedures that can be safely performed in the office are limited to such procedures as removal of lost IUDs, biopsy of focal lesions, removal of small polyps and tubal occlusion procedures. Expanded manipulations and cervical interventions such as the division of extensive intrauterine adhesions or uterine septa, removal of submucous leiomyomas or endometrial ablation are more safely and effectively performed under regional or general anesthesia and, in some instances, with concomitant laparoscopy.

Office hysteroscopy is a simple procedure that can be undertaken in a short period of time with minimal morbidity and inconvenience to the patient. It is important to select the patient appropriately and to schedule the examination during the follicular phase once menstruation is completed (Figures 6.6–6.8). In postmenopausal patients, the procedure can be performed when there is no bleeding. When plastic cannulas activated by suction are used for endometrial sampling, the combined procedures offer an excellent method for evaluation of patients with abnormal uterine bleeding, particularly when no focal pathology is found that requires selective, targeted biopsies. This method of evaluation is useful in premeno-

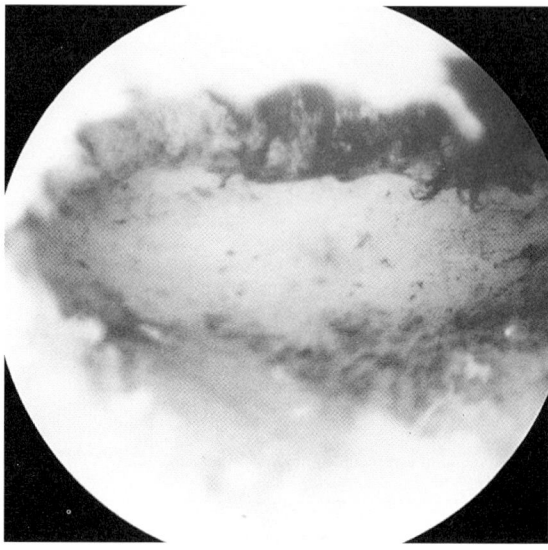

Figure 6.7 Hysteroscopic view of the uterine cavity in the secretory phase

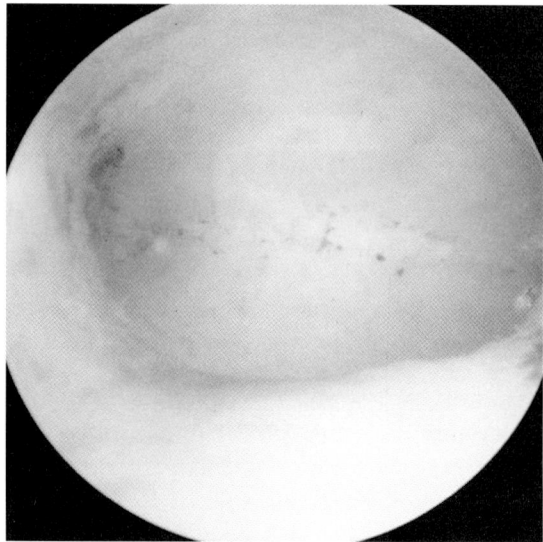

Figure 6.6 Hysteroscopic view of the uterine cavity in the early follicular phase

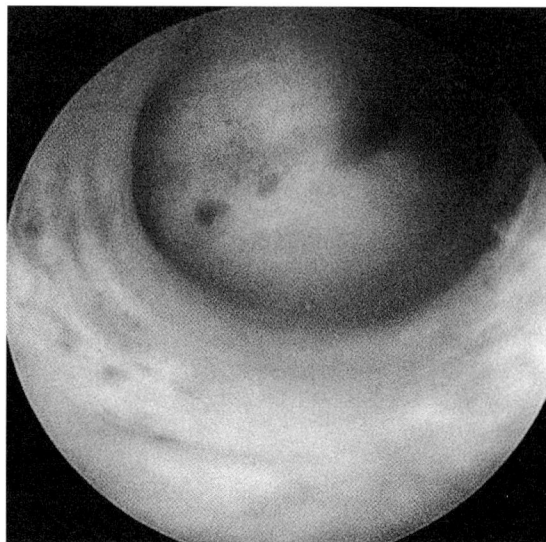

Figure 6.8 Hysteroscopic view of the uterine cavity in the postmenopausal woman shows atrophic endometrium

pausal patients unresponsive to hormonal therapy and particularly peri- and postmenopausal patients with abnormal bleeding.

Practical points for office hysteroscopy

Although the procedure of hysteroscopy is relatively simple, an important factor is to decrease patient anxiety and concerns by adequate instruction. Usually, a nurse or an assistant can describe hysteroscopy to the patient in lay terms and help also with the informed consent. Patients should be put at ease as much as possible by having the simplicity and rationality of the procedure explained. Furthermore, the use of a video system helps to explain findings. While a paracervical block is being performed, the patient should be kept informed as regards each step of the procedure. Ideally, an electrically driven examining table should be used to tilt or elevate the patient as required. A pelvic examination should be performed to determine the size of the uterus and its orientation. Once the speculum is placed to expose the cervix, the vagina and vulva are disinfected. Before any manipulation of the cervix is attempted, a paracervical block should be performed and a tenaculum applied to the anterior lip of the cervix. The hysteroscope is introduced and the findings explained to the patient observing the video screen. Should a Vabra-type aspiration biopsy be required, the procedure should also be explained to the patient. Occasionally, patients may require a non-steroidal anti-inflammatory agent following suction aspiration to relieve uterine cramps.

Office procedures should be simple, expeditious and comfortable to the patient to achieve the full value of these procedures – decreasing expense and inconvenience to the patient and physician, and permitting better utilization of resources.

It is important, therefore, to have the appropriate instrumentation displayed and a special electrically driven table to move the patient into position without difficulty, with local anesthesia if required, a knowledgeable assistant, appropriate informed consent, and equipment for treatment of hypotension or other unwanted side effects or problems requiring resuscitation measures.

Correlation of diagnostic hysteroscopy with hysterosalpingography, vaginal ultrasound and fluid-enhanced sonography

Hysterosalpingography remains the initial screening method for evaluation of the uterine cavity and Fallopian tubes in infertile patients as it provides useful information regarding Fallopian tube anatomy and patency. The information derived from the hysterosalpingogram is particularly useful when normal findings are obtained. When the hysterosalpingogram reveals abnormalities, endoscopy becomes mandatory to confirm or rectify the abnormal picture. Indeed, around 30–40% of abnormal hysterographic findings may not be confirmed by direct visualization of the uterine cavity as the abnormalities may be due to debris, blood clots, mucus or transient distortion of the uterine cavity during performance of the procedure itself.

As only topography is evaluated by endoscopy, ultrasonography complements endoscopic evaluation by providing information about the uterine walls, indicating not only their thickness, but also the presence or absence of intramural or submucous leiomyomas. If central lesions are suspected of being polyps, or leiomyomas are encountered, additional evaluation may be obtained by injection of small quantities of fluid into the uterine cavity as contrast. This permits evaluation of any lesion that is intracavitary and reveals its extension into the uterine wall. Fluid-enhanced sonography does not permit either a panoramic view or anatomical evaluation of intrauterine lesions.

The blood flow of vascular structures such as myomas and polyps can be evaluated by Doppler ultrasonography to better understand their anatomy, physiology and malignant potential. This method, although promising, remains under evaluation.

Magnetic resonance imaging (MRI) is useful in selected patients, particularly those harboring lesions not accurately evaluated by sonography such as adenomyosis, and for uterine evaluation of obese women, particularly when vaginal / abdominal sonography is unsuccessful.

Selected bibliography

Barbot J, Parent B, Dubuisson JB. Contact hysteroscopy: Another method of endoscopic examination of the uterine cavity. *Am J Obstet Gynecol* 1980;136:721

Bibbo M, Kleuskens L, Azizi F, *et al*. Accuracy of three sampling techniques for the diagnosis of endometrial cancer and hyperplasias. *J Reprod Med* 1982;27:622

Burnett JE. Hysteroscopy-controlled curettage for endometrial polyps. *Obstet Gynecol* 1964; 24:621

Englund SE, Ingelman-Sundberg A, Westin B. Hysteroscopy in diagnosis and treatment of uterine bleeding. *Gynecologia* 1957;143:217

Font-Sastre V, Carabias J, Bonilla-Musoles F, Pellicer A. Office hysteroscopy with small-calibre instruments. *Acta Europaea Fertilitatis* 1986;17:427

Goldchmit ZK, Blickstein I, Caspi B, Dgani R. The accuracy of endometrial Pipelle sampling with and without sonographic measurement of endometrial thickness. *Obstet Gynecol* 1993; 82:727

Goldrath MH, Sherman AI. Office hysteroscopy and suction curettage: Can we eliminate the hospital diagnostic D & C. *Am J Obstet Gynecol* 1985;152:220

Gribb JJ. Hysteroscopy. An aid in gynecologic diagnosis. *Obstet Gynecol* 1960;15:593

Hamou J. Microhysteroscopy: a new procedure and its original applications in gynecology. *J Reprod Med* 1981;26:375

Karacz B. Office hysteroscopy. In Siegler AM, Lindemann HJ, eds. *Hysteroscopy: Principles and Practice*. Philadelphia, London, New York: JB Lippincott, 1984:106–7

Novak E. A suction-curette apparatus for endometrial biopsy. *J Am Med Assoc* 1935; 104:1497

Parent B, Guedj H, Barbot J, Nodarian P. In Meloine SA, ed. *Panoramic Hysteroscopy*. (English translation.) Baltimore: Williams & Wilkins, 1985

Rodriguez GC, Yakub N, King ME. A comparison of the Pipelle device and Vabra aspiration as measured by endometrial denudation in hysterectomy specimens: The Pipelle device samples significantly less of the endometrial surface than the Vabra aspirator. *Am J Obstet Gynecol* 1993;168:55

Stock RJ, Kanbour A. Prehysterectomy curettage. *Obstet Gynecol* 1975;45:537

Valle RF. Hysteroscopic evaluation of patients with abnormal uterine bleeding. *Surg Gynecol Obstet* 1981;153:521

Valle RF. Hysteroscopy. In Garcia CR, Mastroianni L, Amelar RD, Dubin L, eds. *Current Therapy of Infertility.* Toronto, Philadelphia: BC Decker Inc., 1988:9–12

Valle RF. Future growth and development of hysteroscopy. In DeCherney AH, ed. *Hysteroscopy.* Philadelphia, London, Toronto, Montreal, Sydney, Tokyo: WB Saunders, 1988

Word B, Gravlee LC, Wideman GL. The fallacy of simple uterine curettage. *Obstet Gynecol* 1958;12:642

7 Therapeutic hysteroscopy

Whether using local, regional or general anesthesia, the technique of operative or therapeutic hysteroscopy is similar to that of diagnostic hysteroscopy except that the endoscopes are larger, usually 7–8 mm in outer diameter and, thus, usually require cervical dilatation. The uterine cavity is distended with low-viscosity fluids and, depending on the procedure, a medium with or without electrolytes is selected. When a tight and difficult-to-dilate cervical canal is encountered, an obturator attached to the outer sheath of the hysteroscope is used for the initial introduction, permitting insertion as far as the cervical os. The obturator is removed, and replaced by the telescope and bridge. When low-viscosity fluids are used for uterine distention, a polyethylene catheter 2.4 mm in outer diameter and 1.6 mm in inner diameter is introduced to the end of the hysteroscope before distention begins (Figure 7.1). The fluid under pressure

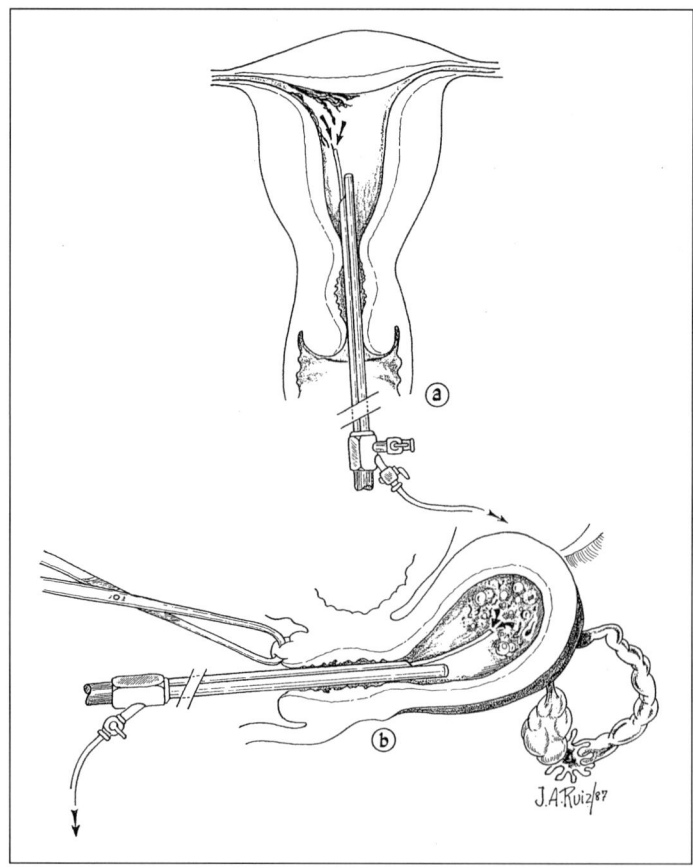

Figure 7.1 Flushing the uterus through a polyethylene catheter

is allowed to enter the uterine cavity, permitting siphoning of the fluid through the polyethylene catheter.

When the distending medium exiting through the polyethylene catheter from the uterine cavity is clear of detritus, debris and blood clots, intrauterine visualization can begin. Targeted aspiration of selected areas of the uterine cavity is then performed with the polyethylene catheter to permit complete and unopposed visualization. If the operative hysteroscope has only one operating channel, the polyethylene catheter is removed to allow ancillary instruments to be inserted. Videocameras can be adapted for attachment to the ocular portion of the hysteroscope before insertion into the uterine cavity after adjustment for uniform color and a focused image. The correct orientation of the hysteroscope before insertion is with the fiberoptic light cable facing downwards, indicating that the viewing telescope is facing upwards. The camera is kept in position without rotation; if rotation is required, only the hysteroscope should be rotated to observe the lateral aspects of the uterine cavity and tubal openings. When laparoscopy is used to monitor intrauterine surgery or for other reasons, the laparoscope is inserted first to allow uterine manipulation such as cervical dilatation or introduction of the hysteroscope aided by the laparoscopic view. To monitor hysteroscopic surgery, it is helpful to dim the light of the laparoscope to permit hysteroscopic illumination through the uterine wall. Innovations in instruments, light sources, videocameras, ancillary instrumentation and energy sources such as laser and electrosurgery have increased the therapeutic uses of hysteroscopy.

Targeted biopsy

Among the therapeutic applications of hysteroscopy (Table 7.1) are targeted biopsies. Biopsies of the endometrium are initially obtained with suction devices, particularly of the Vabra type, to remove as much endometrial tissue as possible. This method has proved especially helpful in the evaluation of patients who have abnormal uterine bleeding and extensive areas of endometrium that need to be biopsied. However, when focal lesions of endometrium are present particularly at the uterotubal cornua and/or confined to polyps, or should submucous leiomyomas be present, these latter conditions may not be correctly diagnosed. Visual appraisal of the uterine cavity can provide accurate targeted biopsies of focal lesions that may be missed by the mechanical or suction devices available today. Specifically, endometrial polyps can easily be detected and extracted, and focal areas of endometrium biopsied directly, particularly those located at the uterotubal cornua where they can be easily missed by blind methods of evaluation. Endometrial lesions suspected of malignancy can be visually evaluated and a directed biopsy of an abnormal area performed. With the currently available hysteroscopic ancillary biopsy instruments, only small portions can be obtained; it is therefore necessary to take several samples of the same area to have adequate tissue for histopathological evaluation.

Table 7.1 Therapeutic applications of hysteroscopy

Targeted biopsy

Removal of endometrial polyps

Removal of submucous leiomyomas

Division of uterine septa

Removal of 'lost' intrauterine devices and other foreign bodies

Lysis of intrauterine adhesions

Endometrial ablation (laser, electrosurgery)

Tubal cannulation (tubal obstruction, etc.)

Chorionic villus sampling

Tubal occlusion (electrocoagulation, cryocoagulation, chemical, mechanical)

Removal of endometrial polyps and submucous leiomyomas

In the past, blind methods of evaluation and treatment were used when attempting the removal of polyps; forceps were introduced and opened blindly in the uterine cavity in an attempt to grasp a polyp. Such maneuvers were sometimes frustrating and inadequate. The visual appraisal of the uterine cavity provided by the hysteroscope offers an excellent method for the removal of polyps, particularly pedunculated polyps, which can be transected and removed in their totality (Figure 7.2). Sessile polyps can be also removed in this manner and the base treated by suction curettage. The resectoscope is particularly useful for removing this type of polyp as the base can easily be resected in its totality to avoid recurrences. Whatever method is chosen for removal, it is important to ensure that the entire polyp has been removed and this can only be confirmed visually by hysteroscopy. There are several alternatives for the removal of polyps, including blind attempts with a curette or polyp forceps once the polyp has been diagnosed and located.

Uterine leiomyomas are common neoplastic disorders that often require surgical treatment, particularly if they are submucous (Figures 7.3 and 7.4). Submucous myomas may invade the uterine wall virtually in their

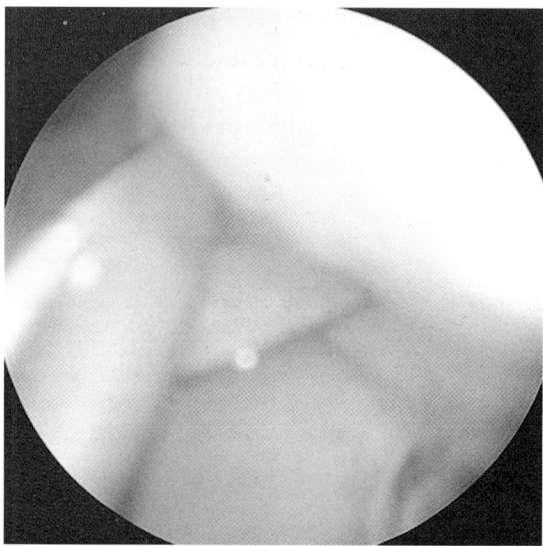

Figure 7.2 Hysteroscopic removal of a pedunculated submucous myoma using semirigid scissors

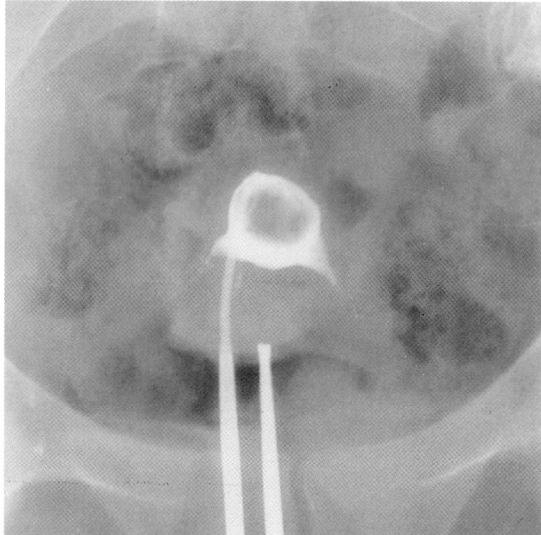

Figure 7.3 Hysterogram showing a uterine cavity deformed by a submucous tumor

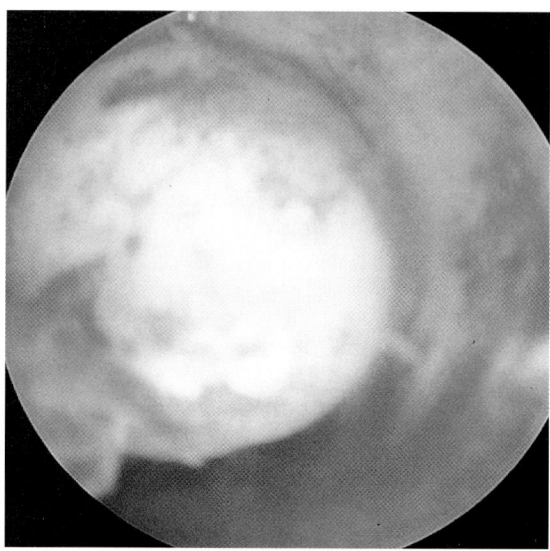

Figure 7.4 Hysteroscopic view of a submucous leiomyoma

totality and show, like an iceberg, only a small tip of myoma in the cavity. This type of myoma cannot be treated endoscopically and may even require a hysterotomy with uterine reconstruction, if symptomatic.

No blind method is useful in the treatment of submucous leiomyomas. Removal of these tumors must be accomplished via endoscopes, which require more experience to use. Several hysteroscopic methods are available to remove submucous leiomyomas (Figures 7.5 and 7.6). When a leiomyoma is pedunculated and no greater than 3 cm in diameter, transection of the pedicle can be accomplished with mechanical hysteroscopic scissors; the cervix can be dilated and the myoma grasped with toothed forceps and removed transcervically. Most submucous leiomyomas are sessile and partly intramural, but most of the tumor is intraluminal. This type of tumor benefits most from resectoscopic shaving of the myoma which causes the uterus to contract so that the myoma that is intramural becomes intraluminal, allowing its complete removal. However, this effect is only noted when the intraluminal part of the leiomyoma is larger than the part that lies within the uterine wall. This can be assessed preoperatively by vaginal ultrasound complemented by fluid injection into the uterine cavity, so-called fluid-enhanced sonography. When the leiomyoma is sessile or has a broad pedicle, the best method of removal is by resectoscopy to systematically shave the leiomyoma from top to bottom until the myometrium is reached. (For more details on the technique of resectoscopic myomectomy, see Chapter 8.)

While concomitant laparoscopy is not mandatory during myomectomy, the laparoscope should be used when resecting large submucous tumors than invade the myometrium deeply or when resection becomes difficult due to location, for example, at the uterotubal cornua.

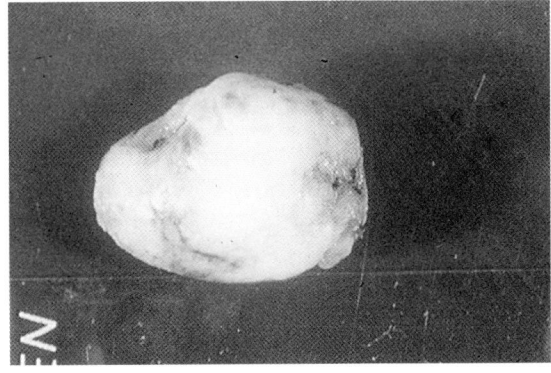

Figure 7.5 Myoma after removal

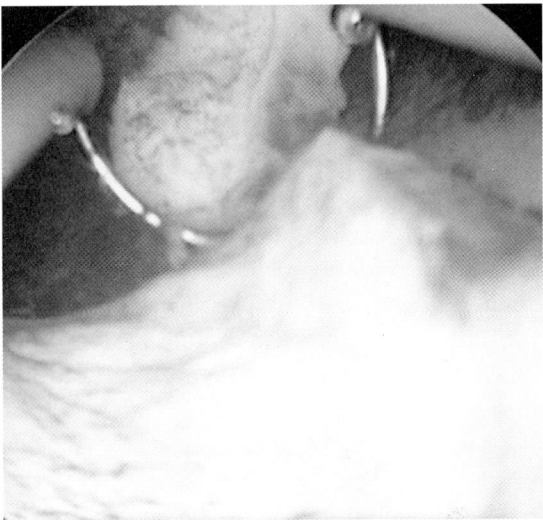

Figure 7.6 Resection of a sessile submucous leiomyoma using a cutting loop

With new advances in the use of the resectoscope, submucous myomectomy has been greatly facilitated and, at present, the gynecological resectoscope is the instrument of choice for these operations.

Results of hysteroscopic myomectomy

The resolution of abnormal bleeding in patients with submucous leiomyomas that do not harbor additional large intramural leiomyomas is impressive: over 95% of these patients obtain resolution of abnormal bleeding provided that the tumor is removed in its totality. Patients who have a portion of the leiomyoma left behind may require a second procedure to complete the myomectomy.

Practical considerations in the treatment of myomas

Uterine bleeding due to submucous leiomyomas may be evaluated by endometrial biopsy and ultrasound to determine the presence of other myomas as well as their number, size and location. In infertile patients, a hysterosalpingogram should be performed to determine the degree of distortion of the uterine cavity and condition of the Fallopian tubes, particularly when the leiomyoma arises from the cornual regions.

If the patient is anemic or there is continual marked bleeding, and if the leiomyoma markedly distorts the symmetry of the uterine cavity, it is useful to treat such patients with gonadotropin-releasing hormone (Gn-RH) analogues to stop the bleeding, and decrease the vascularity of the tumor and its volume. Three or more monthly injections of leuprolide acetate (depot Lupron®) 3.75 mg are required until the hemoglobin and hematocrit are normalized.

The leiomyoma is systematically shaved to the level of the uterine wall. The shavings of myoma are removed as they impair visibility and the uterine cavity is reexamined to determine whether any protrusion of intramural leiomyoma still requires shaving. The tissue is visualized to identify the fascicularis layer of myometrium from the fibrotic myoma tissue, and the cutting loop is activated to cut towards the operator while at all times elevating the leiomyoma from its bed. It is important to monitor the amount of fluid administered and recovered to calculate the deficit, and to attach an indwelling catheter to monitor urine output. If a difficult myomectomy is suspected, the patient should be prepared for laparoscopy.

Uterine septa

Uterine septa cause reproductive failure in about 25% of patients with this condition (Figure 7.7). These patients have repetitive pregnancy losses in the late first trimester or early second trimester with a minilabor, bleeding and abortion. When other reasons for the reproductive failure are excluded,

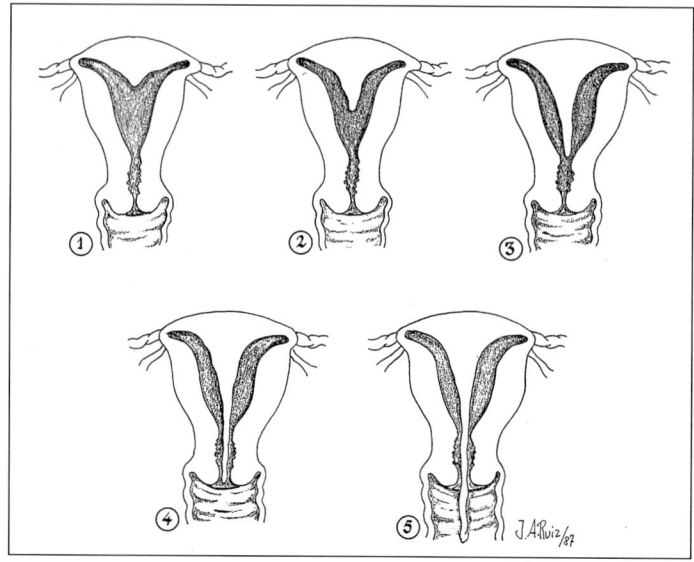

Figure 7.7 Uterine septa range from partial to complete and may include vaginal septation

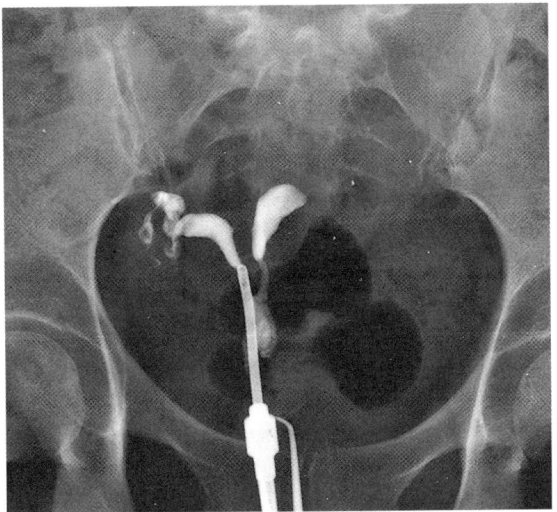

Figure 7.8 Hysterosalpingogram showing a complete septum dividing the uterine cavity

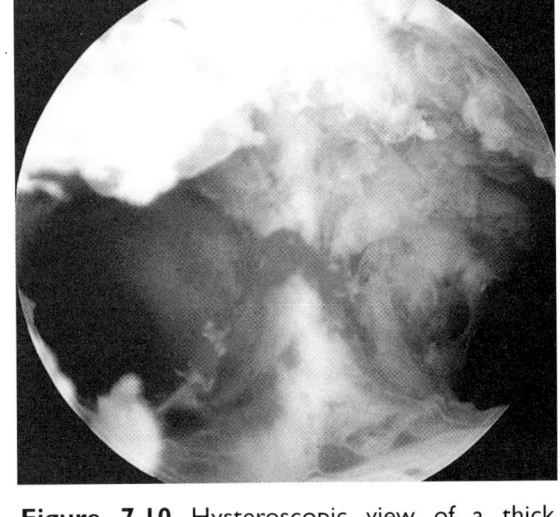

Figure 7.10 Hysteroscopic view of a thick uterine septum

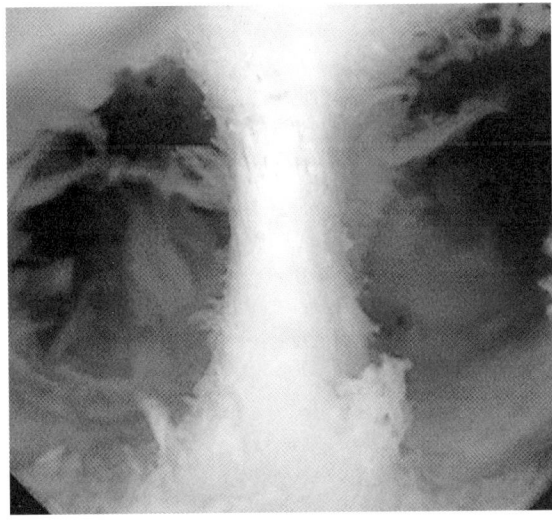

Figure 7.9 Hysteroscopic view of a complete uterine septum

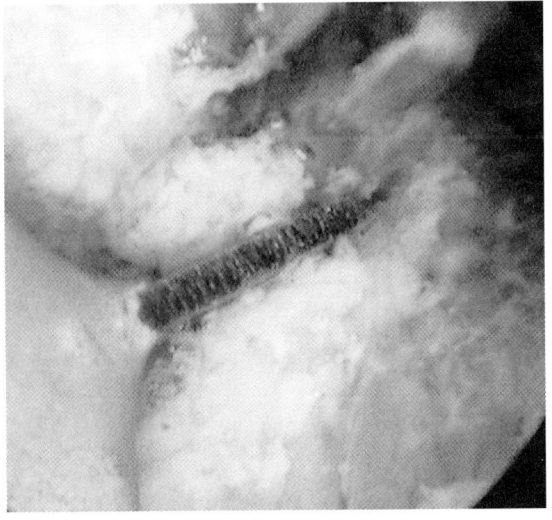

Figure 7.11 Division of the septum using a resectoscope

these patients become good candidates for hysteroscopic surgery.

A thin uterine septum can be divided with hysteroscopic scissors whereas thick and broad septa require a sharp cutting electrode and the resectoscope (Figures 7.8–7.11). Division of these embryological remnants is performed under laparoscopic control to maintain uniform transillumination of the fundal portion of the uterus while the septum is being divided. Once the uterine cavity is symmetrical and both uterotubal cornua are visible, division is complete (Figures 7.12 and 7.13). Care must be taken to watch for bleeding after decreasing the intrauterine pressure by slowing the influx of distending medium. Selective coagulation is performed before the operation is concluded.

Three methods can be used to divide a uterine septum: hysteroscopic scissors; resectoscopic cutting electrodes; and fiberoptic lasers.

Treatment of uterine septum with hysteroscopic scissors

The uterine septum is usually divided hysteroscopically with semirigid scissors (Figures 7.14 and 7.15). The uterine septum, in general, is poorly vascularized; therefore,

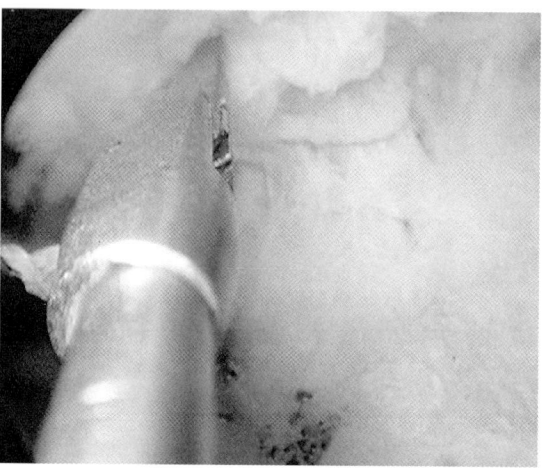

Figure 7.12 Hysteroscopic septal division using semirigid scissors

this technique is useful as division is along the midline, comprising the least vascular tissue and avoiding the anterior and posterior areas where bleeding can occur (Figures 7.16 and 7.17). The hysteroscopic division of a septum is performed with concomitant laparoscopy to monitor the amount of light shining through the translucent uterine wall. Division is performed systematically from side to side until the uterotubal openings can be seen and bleeding is observed at the myometrial junction. Once septal division is complete, the intrauterine pressure of the distending fluid can be decreased; if arterial bleeding occurs, selective coagulation can be performed with a 7-F ball-tipped electrode. A medium without electrolytes such as glycine or sorbitol should be used. If bleeding has occurred, the resectoscope can be used to coagulate selectively each bleeding arteriole.

In general, the semirigid scissors perform efficiently although, if the septum is thick, then rigid scissors may be required. This latter instrument should be used with caution and under a perfect panoramic view particularly at the fundal area. Because flexible or semirigid hysteroscopic scissors

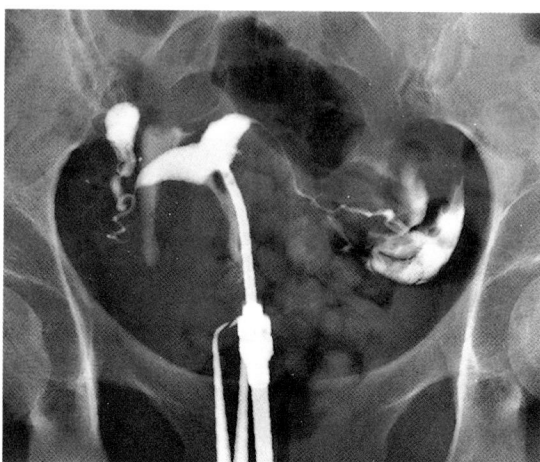

Figure 7.13 Hysterosalpingogram showing a symmetrical uterine cavity following treatment

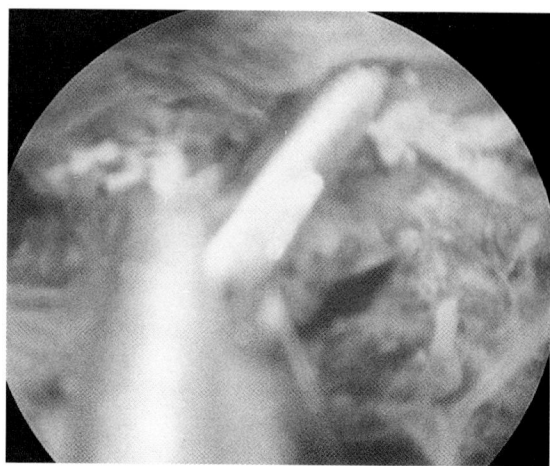

Figure 7.14 Final sculpting of the fundal uterine wall using a semirigid scissors

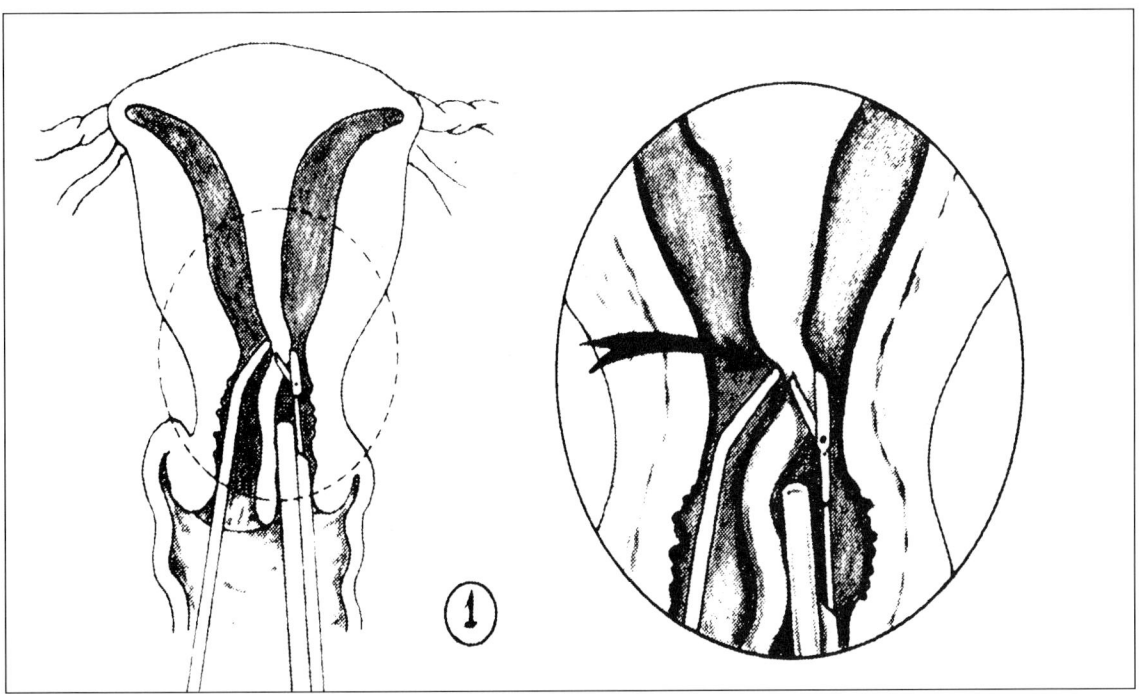

Figure 7.15 Division of a uterine septum extending to the cervix

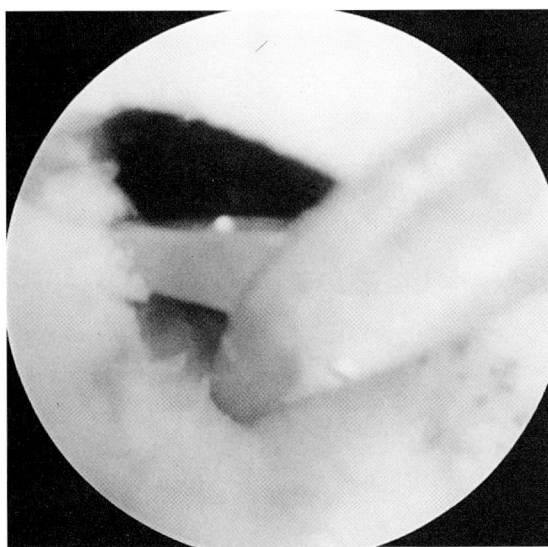

Figure 7.16 Fenestration using semirigid scissors of a uterine septum that extends to the cervix

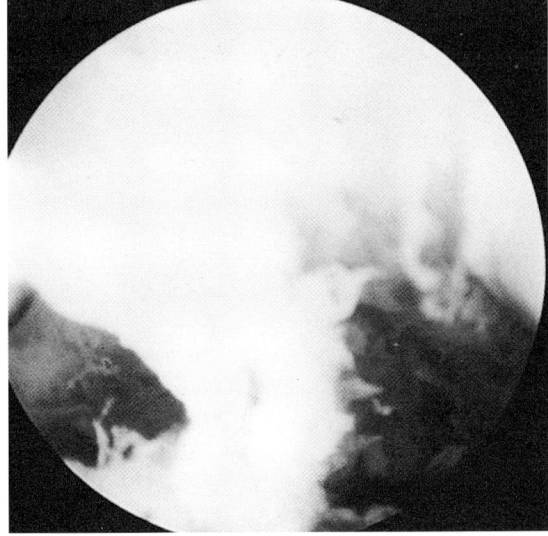

Figure 7.17 Complete septal fenestration is carried out before proceeding with division of corporeal septum

are fragile and may not function properly at all times, a spare scissors should be kept to hand. (Resectoscopic division of the uterine septum is further discussed in Chapter 8, and septal division with fiberoptic lasers in Chapter 9.)

Table 7.2 Advantages and disadvantages of the use of hysteroscopic scissors

Advantages	Disadvantages
Relatively simple	Scissors become dull easily
Quick	Bleeding if not in midline
More applicable to thin septa	Possible perforation
Media with electrolytes	No washing effect unless double-channel hysteroscope used
No energy sources required	Thick septa more difficult to divide

Table 7.3 Advantages and disadvantages of the resectoscope for uterine septum

Advantages	Disadvantages
No significant bleeding	Electrosurgery required (monopolar)
Cuts quickly and easily	Possible peripheral endometrial coagulation
Washing of uterine cavity	Landmarks of myometrium lost
Excellent visibility	Fluids without electrolytes
Advantageous for broad septa	Requires proficiency with resectoscope

Table 7.4 Advantages and disadvantages of fiberoptic lasers for treatment of uterine septum

Advantages	Disadvantages
No significant bleeding	Expensive
Cuts well	Requires special protective glasses
Easy manipulation	Possible lateral scattering
Requires fluids with electrolytes	Requires special maintenance and assistance (Laser Safety Officer)
	Uses continuous-flow hysteroscope

The use of hysteroscopic scissors offers several advantages over the resectoscope, lasers or electrosurgery (Tables 7.2–7.4). Fluids containing electrolytes can be used and the procedure is relatively simple, easy and expedient. When approaching the area of fundus where the myometrium begins, bleeding of small arterioles warns the hysteroscopist that the myometrium has been reached and that the operation is completed. There are, however, some disadvantages: bleeding may require coagulation; the hysteroscopic scissors are fragile and break easily or become blunt; and because no system of continuous flow for hysteroscopy has yet been perfected as with the resectoscope, if excessive fluid is used, significant absorption may occur during the procedure.

Because it is a relatively simple procedure and avoids unnecessary damage to the surrounding endometrium, the hysteroscopic method of dividing the uterine septum with scissors continues to be the preferred method for treating this condition (Table 7.5). The reproductive outcome following hysteroscopic treatment of a symptomatic septate uterus has equaled and even surpassed the results obtained with traditional abdominal

Table 7.5 Comparison of different methods of hysteroscopic metroplasty

Feature	Scissors	Resectoscope	Fiber lasers
Simplicity	++	+	+
Speed	+++	++	+
Hemostasis	+	+++	+++
Applicable to all septa	++	+	++
Evaluation of juxtaposed myometrium	+++	+	+
Cost	+	++	+++
Possible perforation	+	++	++
Required skill	+++	+++	+++
Fluid overload	+	++	++

metroplasty, with a more than 85–90% rate of viable pregnancies. The patient is spared a laparotomy and hysterotomy, thereby eliminating the potential for pelvic adhesions as well as the associated pain, disability and expense. Patients treated hysteroscopically need to wait for only 4 weeks following the procedure before attempting conception, and Cesarean section is not mandatory should pregnancy be carried to term.

Practical considerations in the treatment of septa

Laparoscopy can be performed with a 5-mm laparoscope to monitor the hysteroscopic surgery. The pelvic cavity, uterus, ovaries and Fallopian tubes are systematically observed and the light of the laparoscope dimmed to allow hysteroscopic light translucency through the uterine wall.

In general, semirigid hysteroscopic scissors are sufficient to divide thin septa. For thick and broad septa, the resectoscope fitted with a thin cutting electrode is useful, as this type of electrode can reach the lateral portions of the septum to avoid bleeding. A blend of outputs made up of 80–90 W of cutting (unmodulated) output and 30–40 W of coagulating (modulated) output can be used.

On completion of septal division, the intrauterine pressure can be decreased slightly so that bleeding can be selectively coagulated before the procedure is terminated.

Uterine adhesions

The early follicular phase of the menstrual cycle is chosen in menstruating patients who demonstrate intrauterine adhesions on hysterosalpingography (Figure 7.18). Depen-

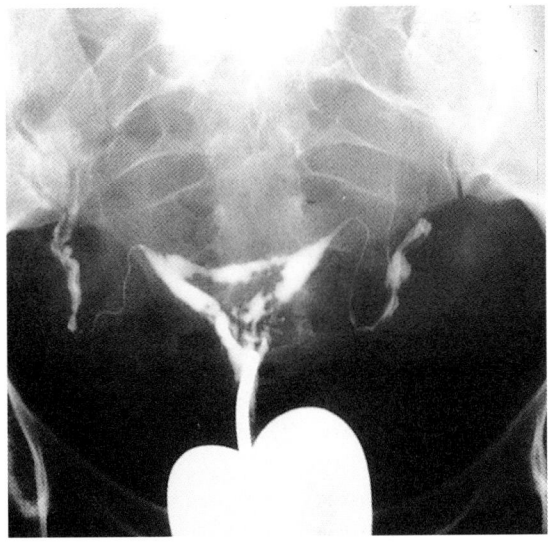

Figure 7.18 Hysterosalpingogram showing extensive central intrauterine adhesions

ding on the extent of uterine cavity occlusion shown by the hysterosalpingogram, laparoscopy is used concomitantly in patients who demonstrate extensive uterine cavity involvement or tubal occlusion. An operative hysteroscope and semirigid hysteroscopic scissors are used to divide these adhesions (Figure 7.19). In many of these patients, the endometrium has been traumatized; therefore, additional trauma or damage due to electrosurgery and laser is avoided by using mechanical hysteroscopic scissors. Fluids containing electrolytes, specifically, dextrose 5% in 50% saline or Ringer's lactate, are preferred for uterine distention. When laparoscopy is performed, tubal patency is evaluated by injecting indigo–carmine dye transcervically. Depending on the extent of uterine cavity occlusion, an intrauterine splint is left in the uterus to keep the uterine walls separated. An indwelling catheter (number 8) is placed in the uterus with 3–3.5 mL of saline solution in the balloon and left in place for 1 week.

Prophylactic antibiotics are used both during and after the procedure particularly when splints are left in place. Cephazolin 1 g is given intravenously during the procedure, followed by cephalexin 500 mg four times a day orally, or doxycycline 100 mg intravenously and 100 mg twice daily orally for 1 week until the splint is removed. To aid in the rapid reepithelization of the uterine cavity, conjugated estrogens are prescribed. Oral Premarin® 2.5 mg twice daily is given for 30–40 days, adding terminal medroxyprogesterone acetate (Provera®) 10 mg once a day orally for the last 6–10 days of the artificial cycle to induce withdrawal bleeding. At the conclusion of the hormonal treatment, a hysterosalpingogram is performed to assess uterine cavity normalcy.

Normal menstruation has been reestablished in over 90% of patients treated for intrauterine adhesions, but the reproductive outcome is related to the severity of the disease. The overall pregnancy rate of 60–70% correlates the extent of intrauterine cavity occlusion and adhesion composition with the reproductive outcome; the more extensive and thicker the adhesions, the poorer is the prognosis. Valle and Sciarra reported that, in 187 patients treated hysteroscopically, removal of mild filmy adhesions gave the best results, with 35 (81%) of 43 patients achieving term pregnancies; in 97 moderate cases of intramuscular adhesions, 64 (66%) term pregnancies occurred but, in 47 severe cases of connective tissue adhesions, there were only 15 (32%) term pregnancies. Overall, restoration of normal menses occurred in 90% of patients and a term pregnancy was achieved in 80%.

Other methods of treating intrauterine adhesions include the use of a resectoscope or fiberoptic lasers (Figure 7.20), although special precautions are necessary when using these techniques to avoid unnecessary damage to the already compromised endometrium. When using the resectoscope, only fine electrodes should be used and the

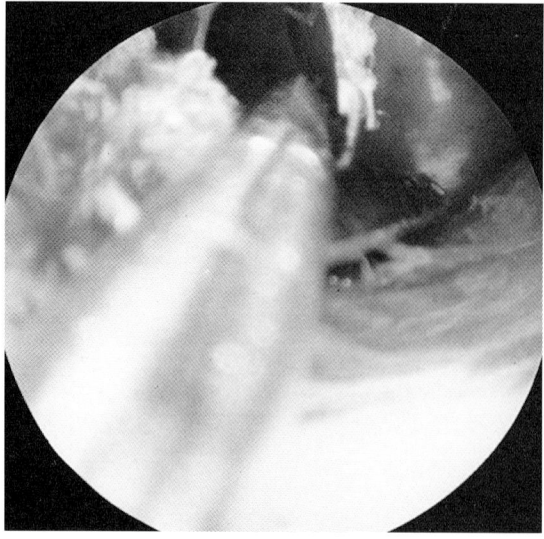

Figure 7.19 Hysteroscopic division of intrauterine adhesions using semirigid scissors

adhesions selectively divided to avoid contact with the surrounding endometrium. When using lasers, only sculpted fibers with thin conical tips should be selected.

The use of hysteroscopy in the treatment of intrauterine adhesions has markedly improved the management of these patients by identifying the type of adhesions present and allowing the selective division of adhesions atraumatically without further damage to the remaining endometrium. The reproductive outcome is better than with the earlier blind methods of treatment. Today, the treatment of choice for intrauterine adhesions is hysteroscopic division. The results obtained with hysteroscopy are related to the type of adhesions found. When adhesions are filmy and focal, the reproductive outcome is over 90%. For fibromuscular and thick adhesions producing moderate occlusion of the uterine cavity, the reproductive outcome is 70%; in patients with thick connective adhesions or total uterine cavity occlusion, the reproductive outcome drops to 25–30%. Therefore, an increased awareness of the possibility of intrauterine adhesions

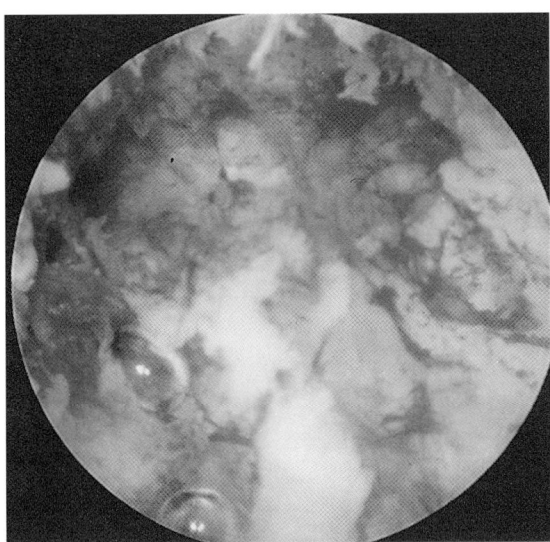

Figure 7.20 Rugged aspect of uterine cavity immediately after lysis of adhesions

following postpartum or postabortal curettage or trauma to the uterine cavity will enhance early diagnosis by hysterosalpingography to evaluate those patients who develop menstrual abnormalities following such trauma to the endometrium.

Practical considerations in the treatment of intrauterine adhesions

The hysterosalpingogram is an important diagnostic adjunct for determining the extent of uterine cavity occlusion, and the condition of the cornual areas and Fallopian tubes. Unless total uterine cavity occlusion occurs, the hysterosalpingogram should be displayed in the operating suite to allow the physician to be aware of the uterine cavity distortion while treating these adhesions.

In general, semirigid hysteroscopic scissors are useful for selectively and systematically dividing these adhesions. Sculpted or extruded fiberoptic lasers with sharp tips may also be used. When electrosurgery is chosen, sharp electrodes can be directed through the operative channel of a continuous-flow hysteroscope to divide the adhesions. The resectoscope is not practical for treating these conditions; the available electrodes do not have tips sharp enough to divide precisely the adhesions without further damage to peripheral areas of already damaged endometrium.

Patients treated hysteroscopically for moderate or severe adhesions require a follow-up hysterosalpingogram on completion of hormonal treatment to evaluate the uterine cavity.

Lost or misplaced intrauterine devices (IUDs)

Although the use of IUDs in the USA has markedly decreased, devices such as the Cu-T® and Progestasert® IUD are still in use.

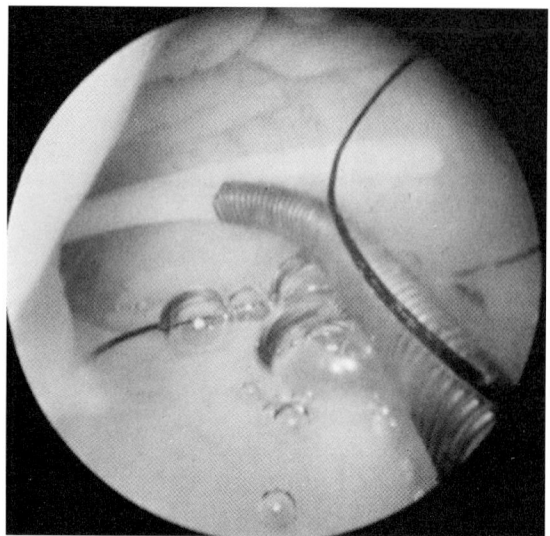

Figure 7.21 Copper-7 intrauterine device with its filament curled up in the uterine cavity

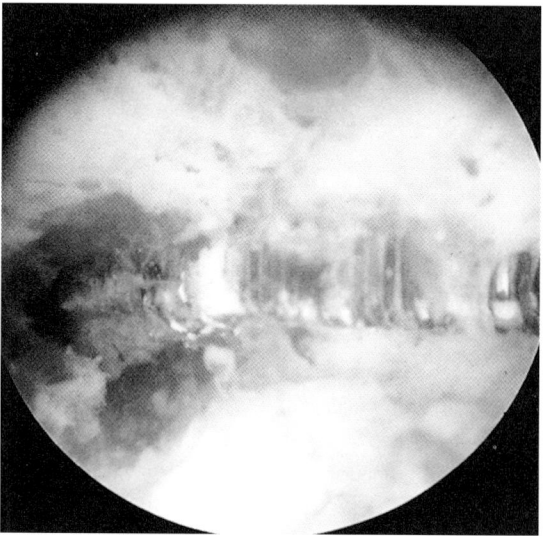

Figure 7.22 This copper-7 intrauterine device is deeply embedded in the uterine wall

Unnecessary radiation may occur when X-rays are used routinely for diagnostic purposes. Potentially traumatic manipulations are often performed in an attempt to remove the devices. In the majority of patients with missing IUDs, the IUD in fact remains in the uterine cavity usually with the filaments curled up in the fundus of the uterus (Figures 7.21 and 7.22). Hysteroscopy is particularly useful not only to detect the IUD and rule out translocation, but also to aid in its atraumatic removal.

After the IUD is located, an operative hysteroscope with grasping forceps is used to grasp either the strings or the IUD itself to retrieve the IUD. This procedure requires only local anesthesia and can easily be performed in an outpatient ambulatory surgical unit or, if the instrumentation is available, in the office.

When the IUD is not visualized in the uterine cavity, a single flat-plate X-ray of the abdomen and pelvis is required to rule out translocation.

Endometrial ablation

Abnormal uterine bleeding is a frequent problem that requires appropriate evaluation and treatment. When the bleeding is due to an organic uterine pathology, the condition must be treated by removing the offending lesion or, when this is not possible or indicated, by performing a hysterectomy. In the absence of organic pathology, abnormal bleeding from the uterus is usually due to either hormonal imbalances or local factors interfering with appropriate hemostasis. Most patients with this type of dysfunctional bleeding respond to treatment with progesterone, a combination of estrogens and progesterone or non-steroidal anti-inflammatory agents and, for those patients with anovulatory cycles who are interested in fertility, treatment for anovulation.

There is a group of patients, however, who do not respond to hormonal therapy and require hysterectomy to treat abnormal bleeding. While a hysterectomy indeed relieves the symptoms, such major surgery causes additional disability, significant expense and inconvenience to the patient. In

Table 7.6 Comparison of different methods for performing endometrial ablation according to complications

Feature	Laser	Rollerball / bar	Resection
Uterine perforation	++	+	+++
Fluid overload		+	+++
contact	+++		
non-contact	+		
combination	++		
Bleeding		+	+++
contact	+++		
non-contact	+		
combination	++		
Injury to adjacent organs	++	+	+++
Coagulation necrosis of uterine wall	+	+	—
Recurrent abnormal bleeding	+	++	++
Pregnancy	+	+	+
Eventual hysterectomy	+	+	+

addition, there are patients at risk of major surgery because of other medical conditions such as coagulopathies, pulmonary and renal problems, and morbid obesity. For these patients, an alternative treatment to hysterectomy is desirable.

Endometrial ablation was introduced to treat abnormal uterine bleeding of dysfunctional origin as an alternative to hysterectomy. Many patients object to hysterectomy unless it is absolutely necessary and enthusiastically choose endometrial ablation. These patients should be assessed to rule out malignant or premalignant conditions of the endometrium and other organic pathology. A hormonal preparation is also necessary to produce thinning of the endometrium to improve the chances of destroying the whole of the endometrium, including the basal layer and the superficial (2–3 mm) layer of the myometrium. To accomplish this, fiber-optic lasers or electrosurgery to resect or coagulate the lining of the uterus can be used (Table 7.6). Danazol or Gn-RH analogues should then be given for 6–8 weeks.

Laser endometrial ablation

This requires a laser that transmits through fluids, is attracted and absorbed by pigments and the purplish color of vascularized endometrium, and penetrates deeply (4–5 mm) into tissue (Table 7.6). Such a laser is the Nd:YAG laser which uses a bare fiber (600–800 μm) with 55–65 W of power. To thin the endometrium and make the surface more uniform, it is important to treat these patients hormonally prior to the procedure, using danazol 800 mg / day for 6 weeks or a Gn-RH analogue, such as depot Lupron 3.75 mg intramuscularly, preferably in two separate injections 1 month apart, to accomplish complete atrophy of the endometrium.

The patient is placed in a dorsal lithotomy position and regional or general anesthesia is used. Because no electrical conduction is involved, the fluids used to distend the uterine cavity should contain electrolytes, for example, normal saline, dextrose 5% in 50% saline or Ringer's lactate.

Ideally, the operative hysteroscope should have a continuous-flow capacity to cleanse the uterine cavity and permit measurement of the recovered fluid. Three different techniques can be used when performing endometrial ablation with the Nd:YAG laser.

Dragging or touching

The bare fiber is dragged across the endometrial surface (Figures 7.23 and 7.24). To ensure that all of the tissue is treated, it is important to treat surfaces systematically, beginning at the uterotubal cornua – the most difficult and potentially dangerous sites because of the thinness of the uterine walls – followed by the fundal area. Once this is accomplished, treatment can then extend to the anterior, lateral and posterior walls as far as the internal os. To avoid cervical stenosis, care should be taken not to treat the endocervical tissue. The fiber should always be dragged towards the operator.

Blanching

The blanching or non-contact technique differs from dragging in that the fiber is held about 1–2 mm from the tissue surface and fired (see Figure 7.23; Figure 7.25). The treated area is thus blanched but, as no farrows or sulci are made, the chances of fluid intravasation are decreased as no additional vascular sinuses are opened. Bleeding does not occur as the treatment is strictly by coagulation. However, as it is difficult to keep track of the areas treated due to the lack of clear differentiation with blanching, in contrast to the dark brown areas left by dragging, it is important to draw lines of demarcation or quadrants in the uterine cavity to avoid leaving behind untreated areas. The technique is similar to dragging in terms of the order in which different areas of endometrium are treated.

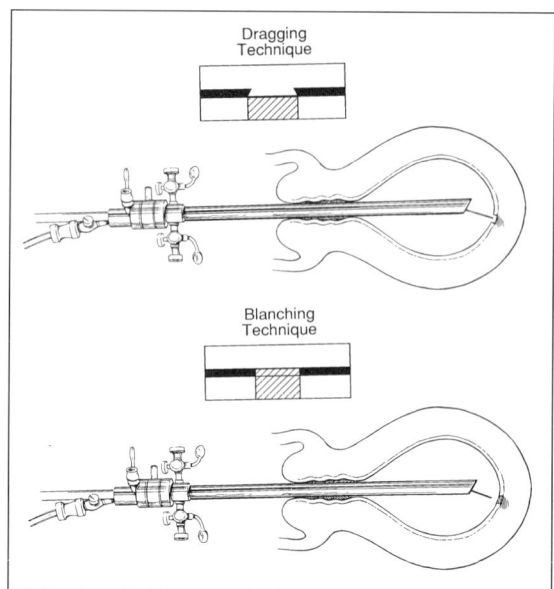

Figure 7.23 Dragging and blanching techniques for endometrial ablation

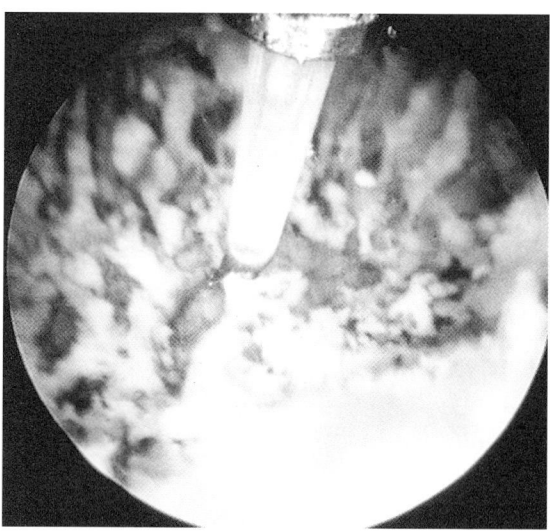

Figure 7.24 Hysteroscopic view of dragging technique for endometrial ablation

Dragging and blanching in combination

Both techniques can be applied, using the non-contact method in the cornual areas and the dragging technique in the rest of the endometrial cavity. This is the most com-

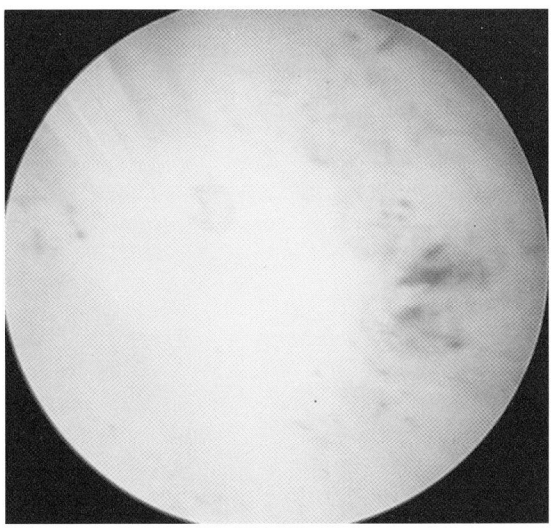

Figure 7.25 Appearances of the endometrium with application of the blanching technique

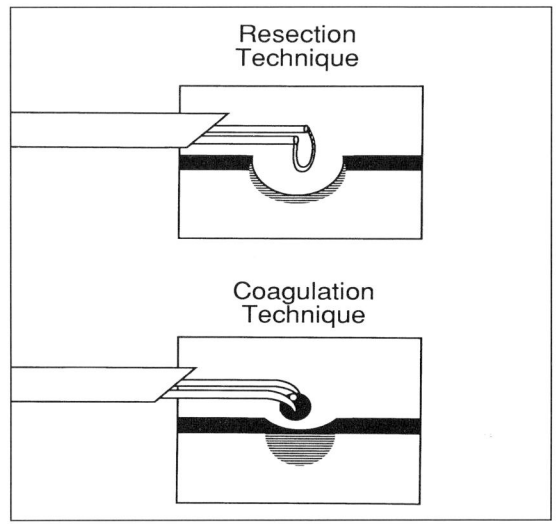

Figure 7.26 Endometrial ablation by resection compared with coagulation using a resectoscope

monly used method of endometrial ablation by laser.

Electrosurgical endometrial ablation

As an alternative to the laser method, electrosurgery can be used to accomplish endometrial ablation by endometrial resection with a loop electrode or coagulation with a roller-ball / bar electrode.

Endometrial resection

With this method, the endometrium and superficial layer of myometrium are shaved with care to ensure that the depth of myometrial resection is 2–3 mm to avoid perforation or excessive bleeding (Table 7.7). Because this technique is more cumbersome and dangerous at the cornual regions, most physicians prefer to do the cornual regions by coagulation (Figure 7.26).

Table 7.7 Comparison of Nd:YAG laser and electrosurgery for endometrial ablation

Feature	Nd:YAG laser	Electrosurgery
Cost of equipment	expensive	moderate
Ancillary help	important	minimal
Duration of procedure	+++	+
Cure rate	excellent	excellent
Failures (bleeding)	< 5%	5–10%
Electrical conduction	–	+
Fluids with electrolytes	+	–
Simultaneous laparoscopy	–	–
Field of view	good	reduced
Ambulatory procedure	+	+

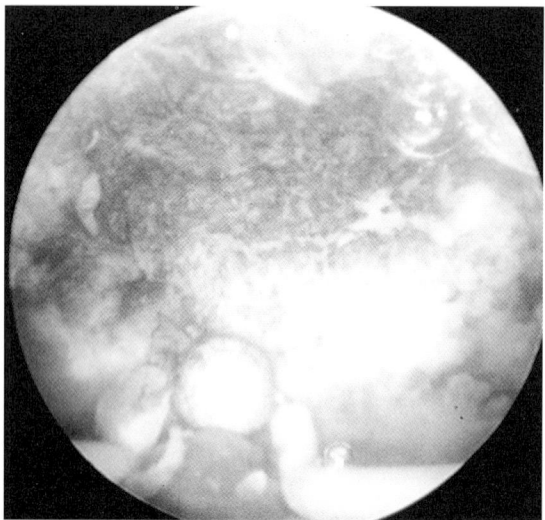

Figure 7.27 Coagulation using a roller-ball electrode for endometrial ablation

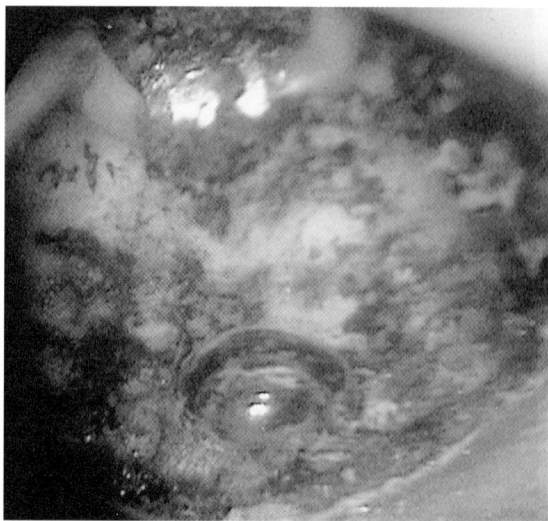

Figure 7.28 Endometrial ablation using a roller-bar electrode

Endometrial ablation by coagulation

Using roller-ball / bar electrodes, the endometrium can be systematically desiccated (Figures 7.27 and 7.28). Although no standard waveform or watt power is used, it is important to obtain results similar to those seen with the Nd : YAG laser. Because electrosurgery is involved, fluids devoid of electrolytes should be used, for example, glycine 1.5%, sorbitol 3%, a combination of sorbitol 2.8% and mannitol 0.5%, or mannitol 5%. A resectoscope 8–9 mm in outer diameter is used.

To avoid high voltages and erratic electrical behavior, an unmodulated or undamped 100–120 W output is preferable. Although coagulating or damped and modulated outputs can be used, they are high-voltage and produce more bubbling when used in the uterus which interferes with visualization. Additionally, a damped and modulated output is more erratic and causes excessive debris to adhere to the electrode, requiring continuous changing of the electrodes to produce uniform tissue coagulation. Studies have shown that a pure cutting or unmodulated output of about 100–120 W is sufficient to achieve endometrial destruction, including the superficial 2–3 mm layer of myometrium.

Endometrial ablation is not a hysterectomy; the patient should be carefully evaluated to confirm that bleeding is not of organic etiology. Other symptoms such as cyclical pain may represent adenomyosis. In addition, the physician and patient should have realistic expectations as the goal of this procedure is not to obtain amenorrhea, but to treat abnormal uterine bleeding.

When these steps are followed, patients can expect an 85–90% resolution of abnormal bleeding. Patients who fail to respond to the procedure may attempt a second endometrial ablation, if so desired, as the results may improve on the second attempt. It is important to rule out organic conditions such as myomas and / or adenomyosis that may increase the possibility of failure.

While patients at risk of a hysterectomy because of medical conditions benefit most from endometrial ablation, other patients with dysfunctional uterine bleeding unresponsive to hormonal treatment may also

Table 7.8 Evaluation of tubal cornual occlusion

Rules out tubal spasm (laparoscopy)

Diagnoses / treats pelvic adhesions, endometriosis, etc.

Rules out distal tubal occlusion

Most infertile patients require laparoscopy

Requires fluoroscopic cannulation if previous laparoscopy normal or contraindicated

If fluoroscopic cannulation fails, proceed with hysteroscopic cannulation (more accurate)

benefit from this alternative should they object to hysterectomy. They should be made aware of the requirements and limitations inherent with this approach. (For more details on resectoscopic endometrial ablation, see Chapter 8.)

Tubal cannulation

Tubal occlusion at the cornual regions can be detected during hysterosalpingography in the evaluation of infertile patients (Table 7.8). Because around 20–30% of these occlusions may be due to temporary spasm, these patients require additional evaluation to rule out such a possibility. Various pharmacological agents, for example, glucagon, ixosuprine and sedatives, have been used to reduce spasm, but none has been successful in eliminating this problem. Therefore, laparoscopy under general anesthesia has been the method of choice. When laparoscopy demonstrates a true tubal cornual occlusion, the patient becomes a candidate

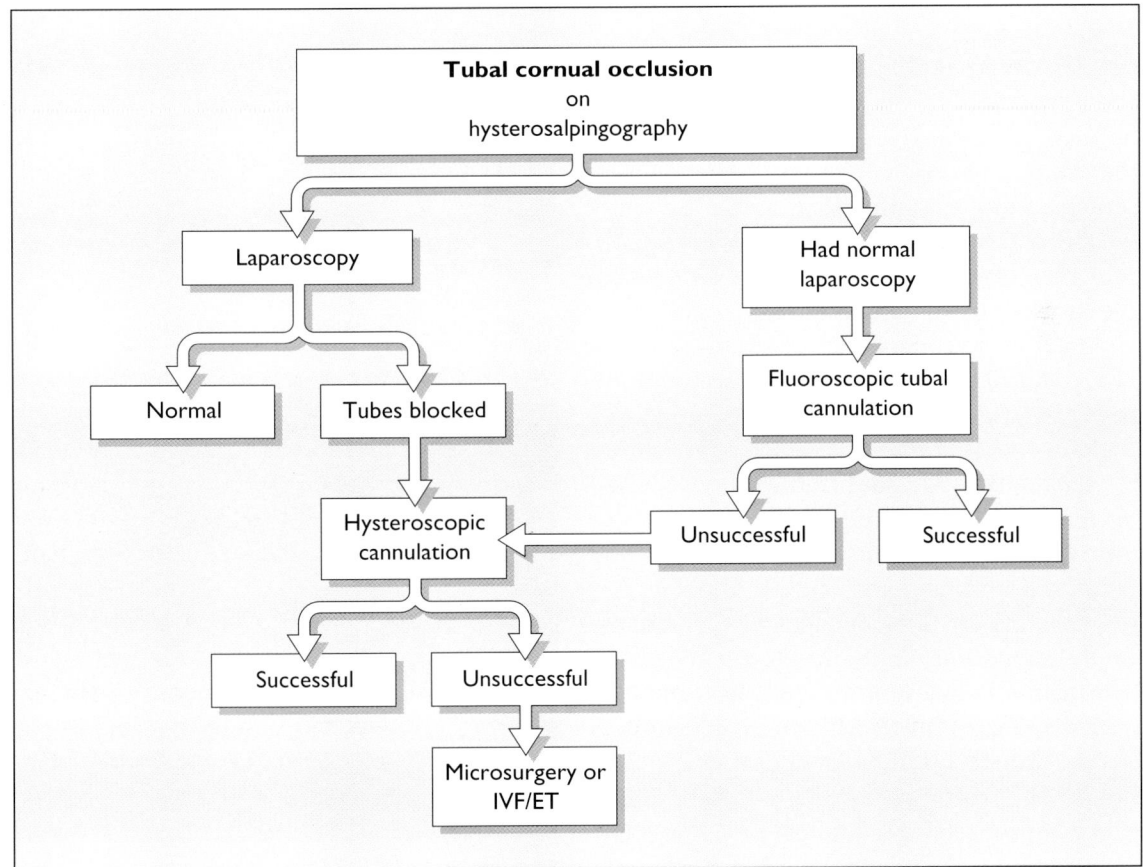

Figure 7.29 Algorithm for evaluation and treatment of tubal cornual occlusion

Table 7.9 Comparison of hysteroscopic and fluoroscopic tubal cannulation techniques

Feature	Hysteroscopy (laparoscopy)	Fluoroscopy
Rule out spasm	+	−
Rule out pelvic adhesions	+	−
Diagnosis / treatment of distal tubal occlusion	+	−
Accuracy	++	+
Invasive (relatively)	++	+
Radiation exposure	−	+
Cost	++	+
Time	++	+
Expertise	+	+
General anesthesia	+	−

for microsurgery to remove the occluded segments and subsequent anastomosis (Figure 7.29). Because frequently the tubal segments removed do not demonstrate true occlusion, the question arises as to the origin of the occlusion. In one series where tubal segments were subjected to histopathological evaluation, it was found that, in more than half the patients, the occlusion was due to tenacious mucus plugs or amorphous proteinaceous material that could be dislodged by probing. This finding confirmed previous clinical observations and prompted the use of tubal cannulation to evaluate and treat these patients.

While hysteroscopic tubal cannulation began in the early 1920s with attempts to occlude the Fallopian tubes transcervically by coagulation for sterilization, it was not until the 1960s that tubal cannulation was introduced by Menken, and perfected by Quinones in the early 1970s. Borrowing from the experience obtained with vascular cannulation and angioplastic procedures, tubal cannulation was initiated by radiologists in the early 1980s with the soft, flexible, coaxial catheters used in angiographic procedures. This method proved to be feasible, effective and reproducible. Because a significant number of patients who have cornual occlusions may also harbor such pelvic

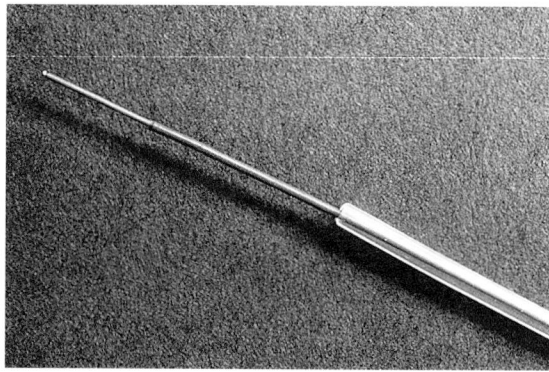

Figure 7.30 A 3-F catheter inserted into a 5-F catheter, with a flexible guidewire in place, is the most commonly used coaxial system

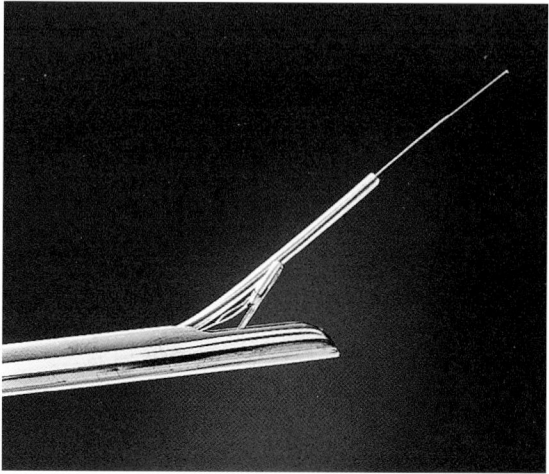

Figure 7.31 Coaxial catheter and guidewire deflected by the lever of the hysteroscope

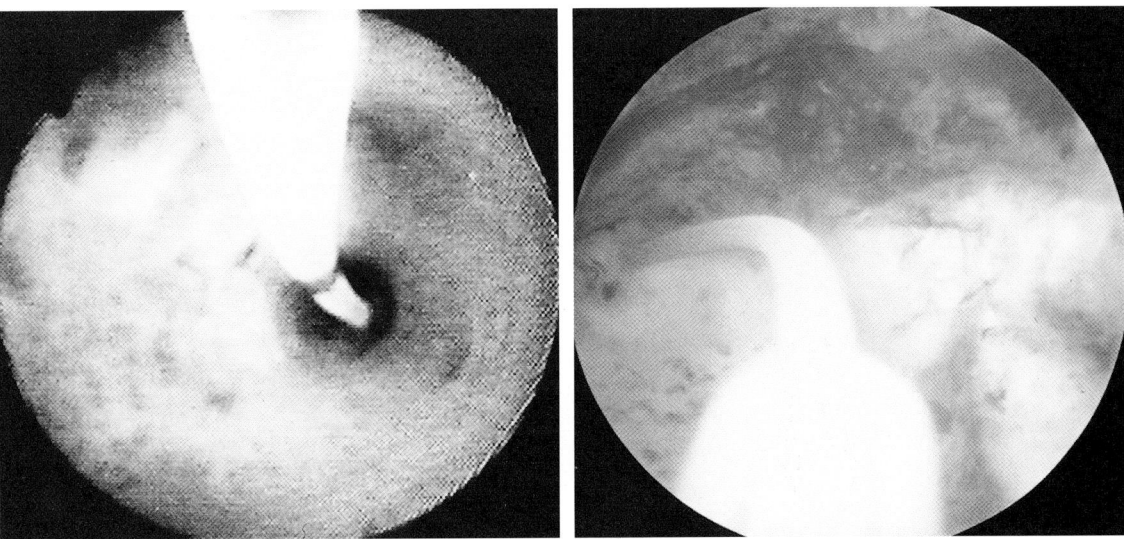

Figure 7.32 Hysteroscopic tubal cannulation using a flexible (left) and rigid (right) hysteroscope

pathology as pelvic adhesions, endometriosis or distal tubal occlusion, the need for laparoscopy encouraged physicians to use the hysteroscope as a more precise and direct method of cannulating the Fallopian tubes with concomitant laparoscopy not only to evaluate the pelvis, ovaries and Fallopian tubes, but also to rule out patients who had spasm rather than tubal occlusion (Table 7.9).

The hysteroscopic method requires coaxial catheters similar to those used during fluoroscopic procedures. A 3-F catheter inserted into a 5-F catheter is the most commonly used coaxial system (Figure 7.30). A soft guidewire that fits inside the 3-F catheter and measures no more than 0.5 mm in diameter is used to find the tubal openings. The coaxial catheters are inserted into the operating channel of an operative hysteroscope (Figure 7.31).

Most physicians use low-viscosity fluids such as dextrose 5% in 50% saline or Ringer's lactate. The coaxial catheters are directed towards the uterotubal cornua and the soft guidewire used to probe the tubal opening without forcing its entrance. The distal portion of the guidewire can be stiff-ened as the catheters are slid forward and, should the inner catheter and soft wire become too stiff, the catheters can be withdrawn to restore flexibility. Once the guidewire has passed through the cornual region, the 3-F catheter is slid over the guidewire, which is fixed distally. When the first portion of the isthmic tube is reached, the guidewire guide is removed and indigo–carmine dye injected through the catheter to ascertain tubal patency as assessed by concomitant laparoscopy. The same procedure is performed in the opposite tube should bilateral obstruction be present.

When there is resistance to passing the guidewire and catheter into the Fallopian tube, the operation should be aborted as this indicates that the tube has a fibrotic occlusion rather than a mucus or proteinaceous plug that can be dislodged by cannulation. These patients should be offered either microsurgical treatment or *in vitro* fertilization.

The results of hysteroscopic tubal cannulation are promising: rates of tubal recanalization range from 70–90%; and intrauterine pregnancy rates range from 45–50%. Nevertheless, the 20–30% reocclusion rate

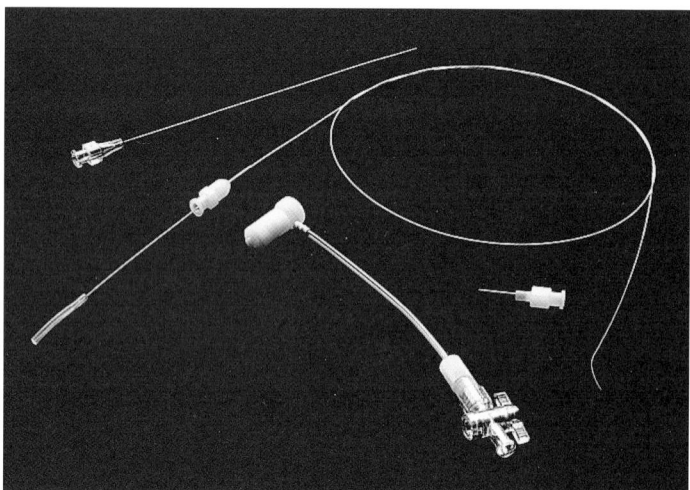

Figure 7.33 Katayama 3-F catheter with guidewire for use with flexible hysteroscopes

and 8% rate of ectopic pregnancy should be borne in mind.

Hysteroscopic tubal cannulation (Figure 7.32) has been found to be an excellent method of selecting those patients who may benefit most from microsurgery, and is the best initial diagnostic method and an excellent therapeutic alternative for patients with non-fibrotic tubal obstructions. Because patients with tubal occlusions may have concomitant pelvic pathology, such as adhesions and / or endometriosis, these conditions may also be evaluated and treated during laparoscopy.

Practical considerations in tubal cannulation

Rigid operative hysteroscopes are best used with coaxial Novy catheters with a 3-F catheter inserted within a 5-F catheter and an intraluminal guidewire < 0.5 mm in diameter. Should a flexible 5-mm operative hysteroscope be selected, the Katayama 3-F catheter with its guidewire should be used (Figure 7.33). No additional coaxial catheters are needed as these 60-cm catheters can be inserted directly into the 2-mm operative channel and selectively bent or steered to a position in apposition to the tubal opening

(Figure 7.34).

Laparoscopy is performed to evaluate the pelvis and rule out additional pathology such as adhesions, endometriosis and / or distal tubal occlusion. Should these types of pathology be found, they can be treated directly under laparoscopic control. If tubal distal occlusion is diagnosed, the tubal cannulation procedure should be aborted as these patients will benefit more from the new assisted-reproduction technologies,

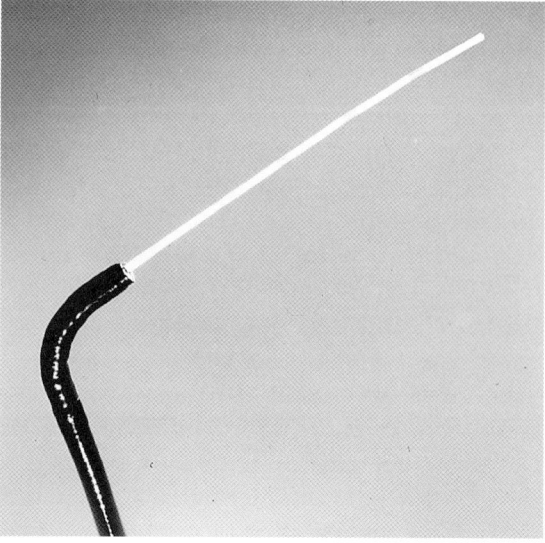

Figure 7.34 A 3-F catheter in place in the operating channel of a flexible hysteroscope

such as *in vitro* fertilization and embryo transfer, than from treatment of bipolar or double tubal occlusion.

Laparoscopy is also performed to rule out tubal spasm, and indigo–carmine dye is injected transcervically to assess tubal patency and confirm cornual occlusion. Although some physicians prefer to perform tubal cannulation under fluoroscopy, there are drawbacks to this approach. Tubal spasm cannot be ruled out and, therefore, some patients may undergo tubal cannulation unnecessarily. Tubal and peritoneal pathology cannot be evaluated without laparoscopy, particularly tubal and / or ovarian adhesions, endometriosis and distal tubal occlusion. Should fluoroscopic cannulation fail, these patients should be offered hysteroscopic tubal cannulation before deciding on microsurgery for tubal reconstruction.

Because manipulation of the Fallopian tube is involved, it is prudent to give these patients prophylactic broad-spectrum antibiotics, such as cephalosporins or doxycycline, to prevent tubal infection. A subsequent hysterosalpingogram will be necessary if the patient fails to conceive within 8–9 months following the operation.

During these procedures, as with any other hysteroscopic therapeutic procedure, a video system is mandatory as it increases the awareness of the assisting physicians and permits sharing the operation with the operating team.

Practical considerations in operative hysteroscopy

The operative hysteroscope should be manipulated with care while maintaining the foreoblique orientation of the instrument. Movements are delicate and the endoscope can be turned clockwise or counterclockwise to see either side of the uterus. Manipulation of the operative instruments, particularly those of the semi-rigid type, should be performed with care to avoid excessive bending as these instruments are easily broken. If bleeding occurs, a polyethylene catheter 2.5 mm in outer diameter and 1.7 mm in inner diameter can be introduced to evacuate any blood clots or debris that may obscure the view. It is important to use this maneuver even before uterine distention begins as dilatation of the cervix usually causes bleeding that may obscure the view when injecting fluids.

Videocameras, when used, must not be turned; only the hysteroscope should rotate. The camera is kept in place with one hand to avoid losing the orientation of the field. If the view is clouded, the lenses as well as the ocular part of the hysteroscope and the camera lens should be removed and cleaned with a dry sponge. Clouding may be due to moisture particularly as the procedure progresses, as fluid may enter the interface and fog the lenses. This phenomenon also occurs frequently when the camera is housed in a plastic hood to avoid contamination. The camera should be adapted to the hysteroscope before the hysteroscope is introduced into the uterus; the colors should be selected while looking at a white cloth, and the image should be focused before inserting the scope. All operating instruments should be placed on the table, readily available for immediate use.

The use of hysteroscopy as a therapeutic tool involves a variety of conditions that can best be treated by this approach. The feasibility of treating intrauterine lesions with minimal invasion brings hysteroscopy to its maximum potential in gynecology.

Selected bibliography

Baggish MS, Baltoyannis P. New techniques for laser ablation of the endometrium in high risk patients. *Am J Obstet Gynecol* 1988;159:287

Baggish MS, Sze EHM, Morgan G. Hysteroscopic treatment of symptomatic submucous myomata uteri with the Nd:YAG laser. *J Gynecol Surg* 1989;5:27

Baggish MS, Sze EHM, Rosenzweig BA, *et al.* Direct hysteroscopic observation to document the reasons for abnormal uterine bleeding secondary to submucous myoma. *J Gynecol Surg* 1989;5:149

Buttram VC, Gibbons WE. Mullerian anomalies: A proposed classification (an analysis of 44 cases). *Fertil Steril* 1979;32:40

Candiani GB, Vercellini P, Fedele L, *et al.* Repair of the uterine cavity after hysteroscopic septal incision. *Fertil Steril* 1990;54:991

Confino E, Tur-Kaspa I, DeCherney A, *et al.* Transcervical balloon tuboplasty. A multicenter study. *J Am Med Assoc* 1990;264:2079

Daly DC, Walters CA, Soto-Albors CE, Riddick DH. Hysteroscopic metroplasty: Surgical technique and obstetric outcome. *Fertil Steril* 1983;39:623

Daly DC, Tohan N, Walters C, Riddick DH. Hysteroscopic resection of the uterine septum in the presence of a septate cervix. *Fertil Steril* 1983;39:560

DeCherney AH, Polan ML. Hysteroscopic management of intrauterine adhesions and intractable uterine bleeding. *Obstet Gynecol* 1983;61:392

DeCherney AH, Russell JB, Graebe RA, Polan ML. Resectoscopic management of mullerian fusion defects. *Fertil Steril* 1986;45:726

Derman SG, Rehnstrom J, Neuwirth RS. The long-term effectiveness of hysteroscopic treatment of menorrhagia and leiomyomas.

Obstet Gynecol 1991;77:591

Donnez J, Schours B, Gillerot S, *et al.* Treatment of uterine fibroids with implants of gonadotropin-releasing hormone agonist: Assessment of hysterography. *Fertil Steril* 1989;51:947

Fedele L, Arcaini L, Parazzini F, *et al.* Reproductive prognosis after hysteroscopic metroplasty in 102 women: Life-table analysis. *Fertil Steril* 1993;59:768

Friedman A, Defazio J, DeCherney AH. Severe obstetric complications following hysteroscopic lysis of adhesions. *Obstet Gynecol* 1986;67:864

Garry R. Hysteroscopic alternatives to hysterectomy. *Br J Obstet Gynaecol* 1990;97:199

Gimpelson RJ. Hysteroscopic Nd:YAG ablation of the endometrium. *J Reprod Med* 1988;38:872

Goldrath MH, Fuller TA, Segal S. Laser photovaporization of the endometrium for the treatment of menorrhagia. *Am J Obstet Gynecol* 1981;140:14

Hassiakos DK, Zourlas PA. Transcervical division of the uterine septa. *Obstet Gynecol Surv* 1990;45:165

Klein SM, Garcia CR. Asherman's syndrome: A critique and current review. *Fertil Steril* 1973;24:722

Lin BL, Miyamoto N, Aoki R, Iwata Y. Transcervical resection of submucous myomas. *Acta Obstet Gynecol Jpn* 1986;38:1647

Loffer FD. Hysteroscopic endometrial ablation with Nd:YAG laser using a noncontact technique. *Obstet Gynecol* 1987;69:679

Loffer FD. Removal of large symptomatic intra-uterine growths by the hysteroscopic resectoscope. *Obstet Gynecol* 1990;76:836

Lomano JM. Dragging technique versus blanching technique for endometrial ablation with the Nd:YAG laser in the treatment of chronic menorrhagia. *Am J Obstet Gynecol* 1988; 159:152

March CM, Israel R. Gestational outcome following hysteroscopic lysis of adhesions. *Fertil Steril* 1981;36:445

Neuwirth RS, Amin HK. Excision of submucous fibroids with hysteroscopic control. *Am J Obstet Gynecol* 1976;126:95

Novy MJ, Thurmond AS, Patton P, et al. Diagnosis of cornual obstruction by trans-cervical fallopian tube cannulation. *Fertil Steril* 1988;50:434

Quinones-Guerrero R, Alvarado-Duran A, Aznar-Ramos R. Tubal catheterization: Applications of a new technique. *Am J Obstet Gynecol* 1972;114:674

Rankin L, Steinberg LH. Transcervical resection of the endometrium: A review of 400 consecutive patients. *Br J Obstet Gynaecol* 1992;99:911

Rock JA, Murphy AA, Cooper WH. Resectoscopic techniques for the lysis of a class V: complete uterine septum. *Fertil Steril* 1987;48:495

Schenker JG, Margalioth EJ. Intrauterine adhesions: An updated appraisal. *Fertil Steril* 1982; 37:593

Siegler AM, Valle RF. Therapeutic hysteroscopic procedures. *Fertil Steril* 1988;50:685

Sulak PJ, Letterie GS, Coddington CC, et al. Histology of proximal tubal occlusion. *Fertil Steril* 1987;48:437

Thurmond AS, Novy M, Uchida BT, Rosch J. Fallopian tube obstruction: Selective salpingography and recanalization. *Radiology* 1987; 163:511

Valle RF. Therapeutic hysteroscopy in infertility. *Int J Fertil* 1984;29:143

Valle RF. Clinical management of uterine factors in infertile patients. In Speroff L, ed. *Seminars in Reproductive Endocrinology.* New York: Thieme–Stratton, 1985:149–67

Valle R, Sciarra JJ. Hysteroscopic treatment of the septate uterus. *Obstet Gynecol* 1986;676:253

Valle RF, Sciarra JJ. Intrauterine adhesions: Hysteroscopic diagnosis, classification, treatment, and reproductive outcome. *Am J Obstet Gynecol* 1988;158:1459

Valle RF. Hysteroscopic removal of submucous leiomyomas. *J Gynecol Surg* 1990;6:89

Valle RF. Tubal catheterization for sterilization purposes. In Gleicher N, ed. *Tubal Cannulation Procedures.* New York: Wiley–Liss, 1992:139–60

Wamsteker K, Emanuel MH, de Kruif JH. Transcervical hysteroscopic resection of submucous fibroids for abnormal uterine bleeding: Results regarding the degree of intramural extension. *Obstet Gynecol* 1993;82:736

Wingo PA, Huezo CM, Rubin GL, et al. The mortality risk associated with hysterectomy. *Am J Obstet Gynecol* 1985;152:803

8 The resectoscope in gynecology

The resectoscope has been used by urologists for around half a century. It was introduced into gynecology in the early 1970s by Neuwirth to resect submucous leiomyomas. Since then, the urological resectoscope has been frequently adapted to make this instrument more applicable to gynecological procedures in the uterine cavity.

Gynecological resectoscopes

In general, most gynecological resectoscopes have been similarly adapted to allow the instrument to be atraumatically introduced into the uterus (Figures 8.1–8.4). The outer sheath in cross-section is round to conform to endocervical canal anatomy; the insulating beak is shorter than that of the urological resectoscope, and the outer sheath has distal fenestrations to permit continuous flow and lavage of the uterine cavity, and to allow accurate measurement of the recovered fluid. The mechanism is the same as that of the continuous-flow resectoscope introduced by Iglesias. Most gynecological resectoscopes

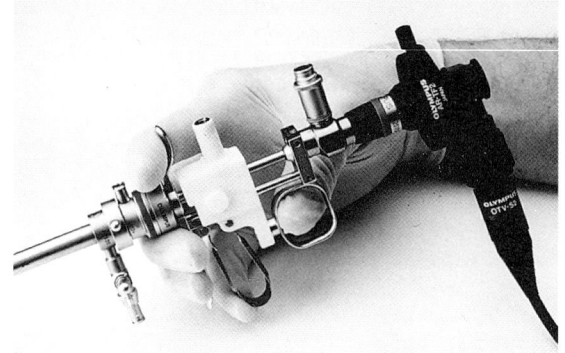

Figure 8.3 An assembled resectoscope with a miniature camera attached to the ocular piece

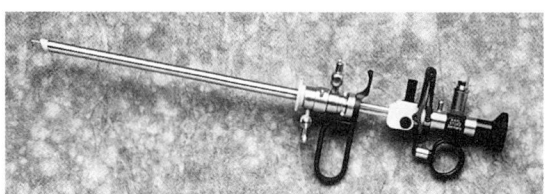

Figure 8.1 An assembled resectoscope with electrode in place

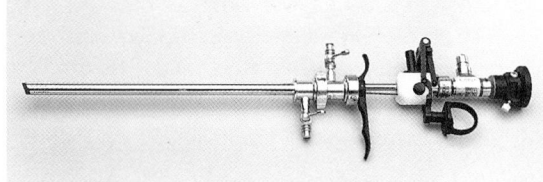

Figure 8.2 An assembled 8-F (4-mm) resectoscope

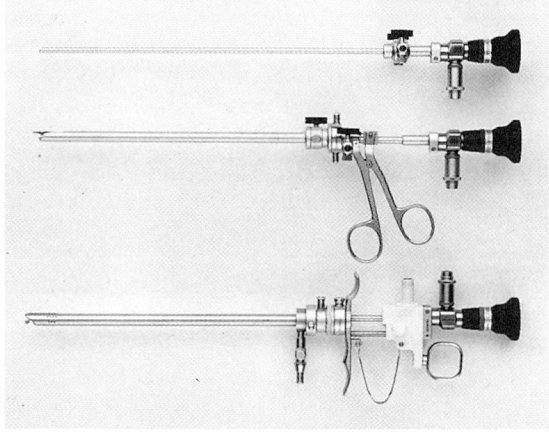

Figure 8.4 Endoscopes used for uterine evaluation include, from upper to lower, the diagnostic hysteroscope, operative hysteroscope with fixed scissors, and resectoscope

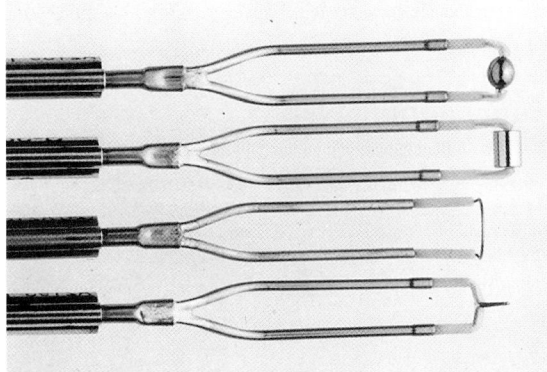

Figure 8.5 Various electrodes for use with the resectoscope

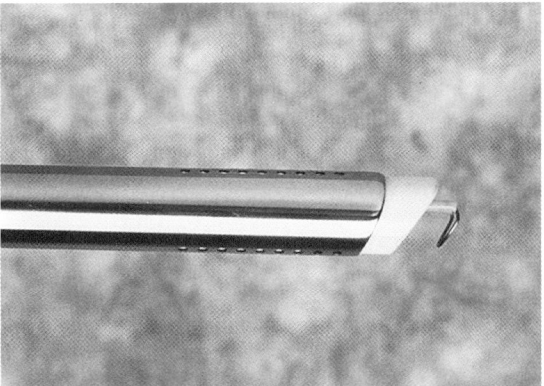

Figure 8.6 Distal end of resectoscope with a cutting loop in place

are 8–9 mm in outer diameter and use loop electrodes for resection, a roller-ball or roller-bar about 3–3.5 mm in length for coagulation, and a curved cutting electrode for division of adhesions or thick uterine septa (Figure 8.5).

Because this instrument requires instillation of fluids and a method of recovery, special tubes are necessary particularly if no mechanical pump is used to deliver the fluids. Large-bore or urological tubing delivers the fluids from 3-L plastic bags and also collects the fluids. Because electrosurgery is involved, an electrical cord is fitted into the resectoscope; different waveforms may be used, depending on the procedure performed, and the outputs may be undamped or unmodulated for cutting or damped and modulated for coagulating, or even a combination of the two (a so-called blend mode).

Because unipolar electricity will be used, the patient should be properly grounded with an electrosurgical plate acting as the return electrode. Only fluids devoid of electrolytes, such as glycine 1.5%, sorbitol 3.5%, a combination of sorbitol 2.8% and mannitol 0.5% or mannitol 5%, should be used. Regardless of the medium, strict measurement of inflow and outflow should be maintained during the procedure and,

periodically, the deficit or non-recovered fluid should be made known to the surgeon.

Applications

Although the most practical and commonly performed procedures with the resectoscope are for the removal of submucous leiomyomas and endometrial ablation, other procedures can be performed, including biopsies of focal lesions that require complete excision performed by a cutting loop (Figure 8.6), and removal of sessile polyps and / or shaving of the base of a removed polyp to avoid recurrences. During the latter, the basal layer of endometrium is also removed.

Submucous myomectomy

The resectoscope has facilitated resection of submucous leiomyomas, particularly those which are broad-based or sessile. The resectoscope is fitted with a cutting loop and the myoma is shaved, beginning at the apex of the myoma until its attachment to the uterine wall is reached. The shavings are not removed from the uterine cavity unless they impair vision: the resectoscope is removed and the shavings retrieved with a polyp forceps or, if necessary, a large-bore plastic suction curette. On occasions, a resected shaving may stick to the loop, thereby obscuring the view; in this event, the bridge either alone or with its inner sheath is removed, cleaned and reinserted without removing the outer sheath. When performing these maneuvers, it is important to remember that bleeding may ensue. Patience should therefore be exercised in that the blood clots and bleeding need to be washed away by the continuous-flow system before the resection is reinitiated. Once the myoma is removed and resection has reached the uterine wall, no attempt to dig into the tissue of the uterine wall should be made. The resection should be almost flush with the uterine wall as the remaining intrauterine portion will become intraluminal due to contractions of the uterine wall. When this no longer occurs, resection can cease. Prior to final removal of the resectoscope, the intrauterine pressure is slowly decreased by occluding the inflow, and any bleeding arterioles should be sought and selectively coagulated with the loop.

While it is easier and faster to resect these myomas using a pure or undamped cutting power output, if bleeding occurs, it will be difficult to perform coagulation unless a blend mode is used. For this reason, a blend output is preferable for myomectomy, using an 80–90 W pure cutting output and a 30–40 W coagulating output in blend-one mode.

When the patient has been properly evaluated by vaginal sonography to rule out other leiomyomas and the intramural components of sessile myomas, the operator will then know in advance how much of the leiomyoma is intramural and how much is intraluminal. This evaluation will help to make a decision as to the approach taken to remove these myomas and avoid the mistake of removing only the tip of the iceberg while leaving behind the greater portion. If vaginal sonography is insufficient, fluid-enhanced sonography may be helpful. Small quantities of sterile fluid are injected transcervically via catheter during vaginal sonography.

Endometrial ablation

There are three ways to perform electrosurgical endometrial ablation: by coagulation; by endometrial resection; and by a combination of coagulation and resection.

The roller-ball / bar electrode is most frequently used for coagulation or desiccation (Figures 8.7 and 8.8). Endometrial resection, including the superficial (2–3 mm) layer of myometrium is common in Europe, but should be undertaken with caution, particularly at the cornua where the uterine wall is thinnest. For this reason, most physicians use the coagulation technique for the cornual regions and the resection technique for the rest of the endometrium. When combining the two techniques for resection of the

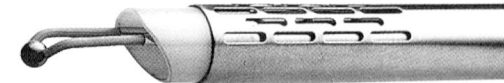

Figure 8.7 Distal end of rotating continuous-flow resectoscope with a ball electrode in place

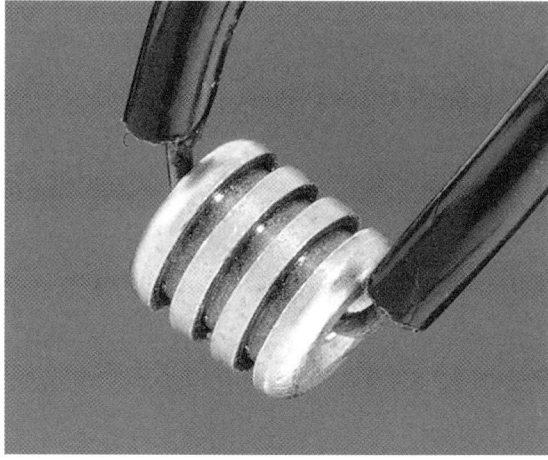

Figure 8.8 Electrode specially designed for vaporization (grooved bar electrode)

entire uterine cavity, particularly in patients who do not respond adequately to preoperative hormonal treatment, superficial resection of the endometrium without involving the myometrium can be performed, with coagulation applied only to the surface.

It is important to ensure hormonal preparation of these patients for uniform thinning of the endometrium before the procedure is performed. In addition, all patients should have a preoperative uterine evaluation and appropriate biopsies to rule out organic pathology, and premalignant and malignant conditions of endometrium.

Either epidural or general anesthesia are the most commonly used methods, although conscious sedation may also be effective in some patients. Although resection is preferred in Europe, endometrial coagulation or desiccation is preferred by most physicians in the USA because it is simple, relatively safe and effective in abolishing abnormal uterine bleeding. Nonetheless, when using the roller-ball / bar electrode for coagulation, it is important to evaluate the patient preoperatively with hysteroscopy and to carry out the appropriate biopsies to rule out malignant or premalignant lesions of endometrium. Furthermore, these patients should receive preoperative hormonal treatment to thin the endometrium, preferably with danazol or a Gn-RH analogue. It is not sufficient to carry out sharp or suction curettage just before ablation as this may not thin the endometrium uniformly and may leave significant amounts of tissue and debris behind, particularly in the form of stumps that hamper coagulation and render the electrodes ineffective by hindering transmission of the electrical power output to the treated tissue. Although resection may not require these precautions, routine evaluation of the endometrium with appropriate biopsies is mandatory.

Although endometrial ablation is an elective procedure requiring previous preparation, occasionally it may be needed for acute bleeding particularly in patients with coagulopathies. In such cases, biopsies should be performed and, if suspicious areas are found, frozen sections should be prepared before proceeding with coagulation. Thus, although bleeding patients can be treated acutely with no previous preparation, and despite the fact that these uteri usually show an atrophic endometrium, relapses may occur. It is therefore important that these patients be frequently followed-up and that they be warned of the possibility of relapse.

Occasionally, a patient receiving endometrial suppression may not be adequately suppressed. Although a thick endometrium may be found in less than 5% of these patients, superficial resection of the endometrium not including the myometrium can be performed, followed by coagulation with a roller-ball / bar electrode.

Other applications of the resectoscope are less defined or require specific modifications (Figure 8.9). These include the treatment of uterine septa with a cutting electrode and the division of intrauterine adhesions. Whereas thin septa are best treated with hysteroscopic scissors, thick broad septa benefit from the use of the resectoscope. However, despite the fact that the electrodes currently available are not designed for this purpose, a thin electrode – preferably bent at one end—is particularly useful for treating this condition as it is able to reach the

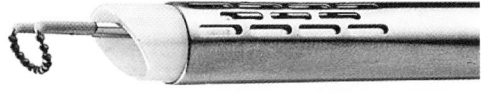

Figure 8.9 Distal end of rotating continuous-flow resectoscope with a roller cutting electrode in place

cornual extensions of broad septa and avoid damage to the endometrium. A forward-directed loop is not as efficient in reaching these areas as is the thinnest possible electrode. When using the resectoscope to divide a uterine septum, the utmost care should be exercised to maintain the symmetry of the uterine cavity during the procedure. Because electrosurgery does not permit observation of the junction between the septum and the myometrium, which may not bleed because of the electrical effect, the hysteroscopist may receive no warning that the myometrial layer has been reached. It is important, therefore, to dim the light of the laparoscope as much as possible to allow transillumination of the hysteroscopic light through the uterine wall, which may reveal to the hysteroscopist areas of possible thinning of the myometrium, thereby avoiding perforation.

Similarly, the resectoscope is a difficult instrument to use in the treatment of intrauterine adhesions as the currently available electrodes cannot be directed to specific areas of the uterus to selectively dissect these adhesions. Furthermore, scattering of the electrical output may damage the already compromised endometrium. For these reasons, if electrosurgery is used to divide adhesions, it is better to use needle-point electrodes guided through a hysteroscope to maximize their steerability and reduce the damage to the peripheral endometrium.

Because myomectomy with the resectoscope is a procedure that predisposes the patient to excess fluid absorption, it is important in these patients to take all the precautions necessary to avoid fluid overload (Table 8.1). An indwelling catheter should be used to measure urine output, and fluid intake and outflow, and differentials or deficits should be strictly monitored. The anesthesiologist should monitor all vital signs and pulse oximetry, and maintain careful measurement of the fluids given intravenously. In addition, regional anesthesia is preferable to general anesthesia. Finally, the electrosurgical unit should have the capability to display the type of waveform selected and the wattage requested.

Basic techniques in resectoscopy

The fundamental components of a resectoscope (Figure 8.10) include: an outer sheath 8–9 mm in diameter; an inner sheath 7.5–8.5 mm in diameter; a supporting bridge for attaching the telescope and various electrodes; a telescope 4 mm in diameter with a 12–30° angle of view; and various types of electrodes, such as loops, roller-ball / bar and a cutting knife (Figures 8.11 and 8.12).

The electrosurgical unit should display the type of waveform selected, whether undamped (cutting) or damped (coagulating). Different blends of these two waveforms and the selected wattages should also be displayed (Figure 8.13).

While various electrical output settings can be used for different procedures, it is important to remember the particular

Table 8.1 Avoiding fluid overload during hysteroscopic myomectomy

With the anesthesiologist, discuss the complexity of the procedure, intravenous fluids, patient's risks

Consider epidural anesthesia in high-risk patients

Place indwelling catheter to monitor urine output

Keep accurate account of fluid deficit (inflow / outflow)

Look for signs of decompensation: vital signs, decreased oxygenation (pulse oximetry), hypothermia (esophageal probe), and ECG

If the deficit is > 700 mL, evaluate electrolytes (Na), status of procedures and patient's condition

Stop procedure if deficit is > 800 mL, electrolytes (Na) decrease, there are positive signs of decompensation, or extended time is needed to complete procedure

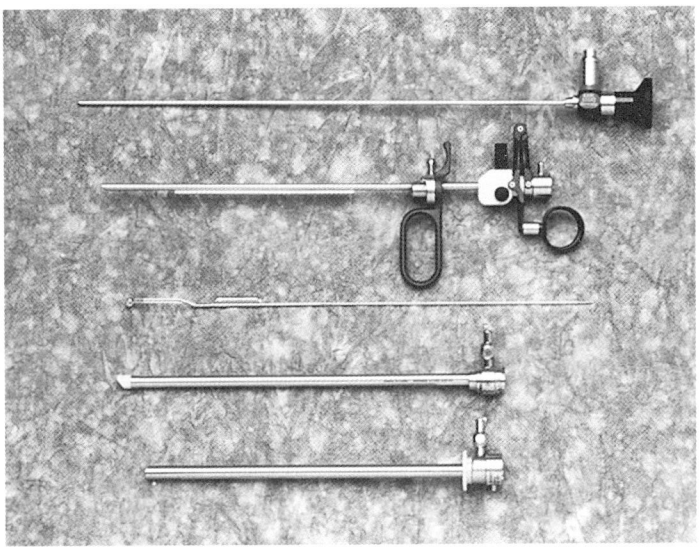

Figure 8.10 An unassembled 9-F resectoscope comprises, from upper to lower, the telescope, bridge, electrode, and two concentric sheaths

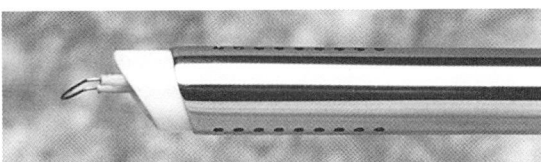

Figure 8.11 Distal end of a resectoscope with a forward-bending cutting loop electrode in place

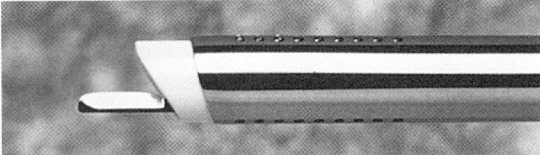

Figure 8.12 Distal end of a resectoscope with a knife electrode in place

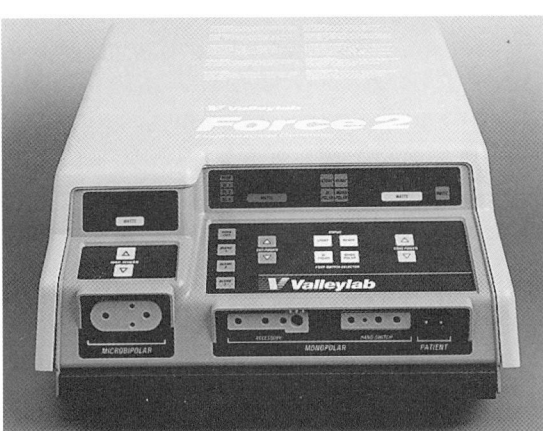

Figure 8.13 This electrosurgical unit is capable of displaying different waveforms

requirements for each of the various procedures. In general, when resecting a myoma, an undamped or pure cutting output may be used as it facilitates shaving of the tumor. However, on occasions, bleeding may occur

and, therefore, it is useful to add a damped (coagulating) output. A useful setting is a blend of these two outputs, using 80–100 W for cutting and 30–40 W for coagulating (at blend one). The myoma is cut by activating the cutting pedal and, if coagulation is required, the appropriate output can be obtained by pressing the coagulating pedal.

While performing endometrial ablation, a specific waveform that can be measured and controlled may be selected. It is useful to remember the effects of the waveform used. An undamped pure cutting output is optimally 100–120 W. This choice of watt power is based on experimental evidence showing that, when a cutting output of < 90 W is used, penetration is somewhat superficial (< 2 mm) and, if an output of > 120 W is used, penetration also decreases, probably due to carbonization of tissue which impedes penetration. Whenever an electrical energy is used, it should preferably be of a low voltage as this appears to behave less erratically than a damped output and produces less bubbling of distending fluid in the uterus.

In contrast, a pure coagulating output of 40–50 W appears to be sufficient for 3 mm of penetration, with the electrode rolled at a uniform speed. If the watt-power is increased to more than 50 W, more debris accumulates on the electrodes, requiring frequent changes to achieve the desired penetration. Furthermore, this type of high-voltage waveform also produces excessive bubbling, leading to pauses during the procedure while the excessive foam caused by the bubbles is evacuated.

It must be remembered, however, that many variables may affect the amount of tissue penetration produced by electrosurgery. Therefore, waveform and wattage, although important, are not the only criteria for adequate tissue penetration. The speed of the roller-ball / bar electrode, the size and shape of the selected electrodes, and tissue impedance also play major roles.

Practical considerations in resectoscopy

The resectoscope should be assembled appropriately, ensuring that the electrodes are well fixed and secure, and that the electrical cable is in place before the electrosurgical unit is activated. It is useful to test the electrical power before initiating the procedure by first touching the relevant tissue – the myoma, if a myomectomy is to be performed, or the uterine wall, if ablation is intended. If cervical dilatation is difficult, an obturator fitted to the assembled inner and outer cannulas may help in the initial introduction. The cervical canal should be dilated to at least the size of the resectoscope or 0.5 mm more to permit easy insertion of the resectoscope through the cervical canal. If resected tissue adheres to the loop or electrode and obstructs the view, the bridge and its attachments should be removed and cleaned. It is not necessary to remove the concentric sheaths unless they also require cleaning. Although the sheaths are not removed, the running fluid should be stopped, by turning the inflow stop-cock, to avoid splashing the fluid onto the floor.

On initial insertion of the resectoscope, it is important to be patient and wait until all blood clots and debris are removed by the continuous-flow system before proceeding with the operation. The dominant hand should always be used to manipulate the resectoscope while the other hand stabilizes the videocamera.

The electrodes should be changed periodically, particularly if they become covered by excessive tissue or are bent. When roller-ball / bar electrodes are used, it is important to have several electrodes to hand which can be exchanged as needed. The removed electrode can be cleaned by the assistant nurse, who should remove the debris with sandpaper and appropriate cloths or sponges.

The loop electrode should not be used for myomas without the electrical output being activated, as it may be easily bent or broken. Loops can be used on soft tissue without electrosurgery for superficial shaving of a thick endometrium or a polyp.

Selected bibliography

Bieber EJ, Loffer FD, eds. *Gynecologic Resectoscopy.* Cambridge, MA: Blackwell Science, 1995

DeCherney AH, Russell JB, Graebe RA, Polan ML. Resectoscopic management of mullerian fusion defects. *Fertil Steril* 1986;45:726

DeCherney AH, Diamond MP, Lavy G, Polan ML. Endometrial ablation for intractable uterine bleeding: Hysteroscopic resection. *Obstet Gynecol* 1987;70:668

Friedman A, Defazio J, DeCherney AH. Severe obstetric complications following hysteroscopic lysis of adhesions. *Obstet Gynecol* 1986;67:864

Hallez JP, Netter A, Cartier R. Methodical intrauterine resection. *Am J Obstet Gynecol* 1987;156:1080

Iglesias JJ, Sporer A, Gellman AC, Seebode JJ. New Iglesias resectoscope with continuous irrigation, simultaneous suction, and low intravesicle pressure. *J Urol* 1975;114:929

Kivnick S, Kanter M. Bowel injury from roller-ball ablation of the endometrium. *Obstet Gynecol* 1992;79:833

Loffer FD. Removal of large symptomatic intrauterine growths by the hysteroscopic resectoscope. *Obstet Gynecol* 1990;76:836

McCarthy JF. A new apparatus for endoscopic plastic surgery of the prostate, diathermia, and excision of vesical growths. *J Urol* 1931;26:695

McLucas B. The resectoscope in gynecologic surgery. *Female Patient* 1990;15:83

Neuwirth RS, Amin AK. Excision of submucous fibroids with hysteroscopic control. *Am J Obstet Gynecol* 1976;126:95

Rock JA, Murphy AA, Cooper WH. Resectoscopic techniques for the lysis of a class V: complete uterine septum. *Fertil Steril* 1987;48:495

Sullivan B, Kenny P, Seibel J. Hysteroscopic resection of fibroid with thermal injury to sigmoid. *Obstet Gynecol* 1992;80:546

Valle RF. Roller-ball endometrial ablation. In Gordon AG, ed. *Endometrial Ablation, Vol. 9, Baillière's Clinical Obstetrics and Gynecology.* London: Baillière–Tindall, 1995:299–316

Vercellini P, Vendola N, Colombo A, *et al.* Hysteroscopic metroplasty with resectoscope or microscissors for the correction of septate uterus. *Surg Gynecol Obstet* 1993;176:439

9 Laser hysteroscopy

Without doubt, the introduction of lasers into medicine has greatly facilitated many surgical procedures, particularly when used with endoscopes. Of the lasers available, the CO_2 laser has been most commonly used by gynecologists particularly in laparoscopy. The CO_2 laser is versatile and can be passed through the endoscope, thereby avoiding additional punctures in the abdomen. Its penetration is well controlled as what you see is what you get, and its shallow effects can be applied with precision without massive thermal damage to surrounding structures. However, its use requires transmission by an endoscope with built-in mirrors and it does not coagulate vessels well nor can it be used through liquid media because of its lack of penetration in fluids. For these reasons, the CO_2 laser is not practical for hysteroscopy. Furthermore, its delivery requires a special system of mirrors to reflect the beam, making it impractical in hysteroscopy. As the uterus must be distended with fluids if gases such as CO_2 are used, the smoke and plume cannot be evacuated without collapsing the uterine cavity.

Fortunately, fiberoptic lasers are available which use small fibers and can be activated through fluids, such as the Nd:YAG, argon and KTP-532 lasers (Table 9.1). Other lasers have recently been introduced, such as the holmium–YAG and the erbium–YAG, and are excellent coagulators able to penetrate further than the CO_2 laser. The fact that these newer lasers can be activated through the hysteroscope and permit operation through fluids makes them another useful alternative for hysteroscopic surgery.

The Nd:YAG laser has been the most commonly used laser for hysteroscopy particularly for endometrial ablation and, with the new sculpted fibers, for treatment of uterine septa and / or intrauterine adhesions. Because these lasers do not involve conduction, the uterine cavity can be distended with fluids containing electrolytes, thus adding a safety factor to prevent fluid overload, which can easily be avoided with the use of diuretics. However, because these lasers are attracted by pigment and reflected backward, the operator must wear either goggles or special filters to prevent injury to the retina. Alternatively, the continuous use of a video monitor may also avoid this hazard. The fibers most commonly used are either not coaxial or are bare fibers that transmit the coagulating effect of the Nd:YAG, penetrating about 4–5 mm in depth and, due to

Table 9.1 Physical properties of lasers used in hysteroscopic surgery

	Wavelength (nm)	Color spectrum	Power (W)	Absorption	Aiming beam
Argon	488–514	blue-green	0–20	Hb + melanin	argon
KTP-532	532	green	0–40	Hb + melanin	KTP
Nd:YAG	1064	near infrared	0–170	tissue protein	helium–neon

Hb, hemoglobin; KTP, potassium titanyl phosphate; Nd:YAG, neodymium–yttrium–aluminum–garnet

Table 9.2 Clinical features of lasers used in hysteroscopic surgery

	Passed through fiber	Scattering	Passes through fluids	Penetration (mm)	Coagulation	Cutting
Argon	+	+	+	1–2	+	+/−
KTP-532	+	+	+	1–2	+	+/−
Nd : YAG	+	+++	+	3–4	+++	+*

KTP, potassium titanyl phosphate; Nd : YAG, neodymium–yttrium–aluminum–garnet
*with sculpted tips

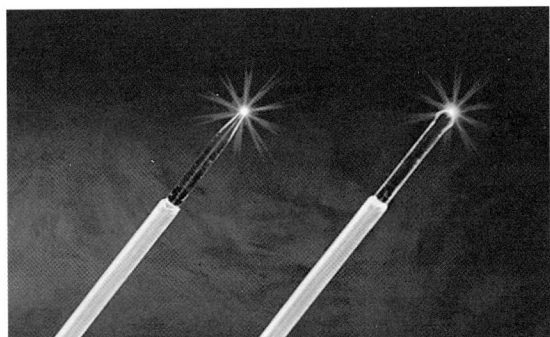

Figure 9.1 Lasers with conical (left) and ball-shaped (right) sculpted fiber tips

the anterolateral scattering effect of this laser, forming craters in the tissue. This is a coagulating laser and is most useful for endometrial ablation. Sculpted fibers concentrate the energy of the laser, depending on the shape of the tip. A conical tip converts the laser into a light scalpel, and reduces the scattering and thermal damage while cutting, whereas a ball-shaped tip can be used for coagulation (Figure 9.1).

The argon and KTP-532 lasers are less used in gynecology. They can penetrate 1–2 mm into tissue and produce less scattering than the Nd : YAG laser (Figure 9.2). They can be used in contact with tissue or fired without touching the tissue and change their coagulating or cutting ability according to their distance from the tissue (Table 9.2).

Clinical applications

The hysteroscopic procedures most frequently performed with fiberoptic lasers are endometrial ablation and removal of pedunculated submucous leiomyomas (Figure 9.3). Endometrial ablation usually requires use of the Nd : YAG laser because of its capacity

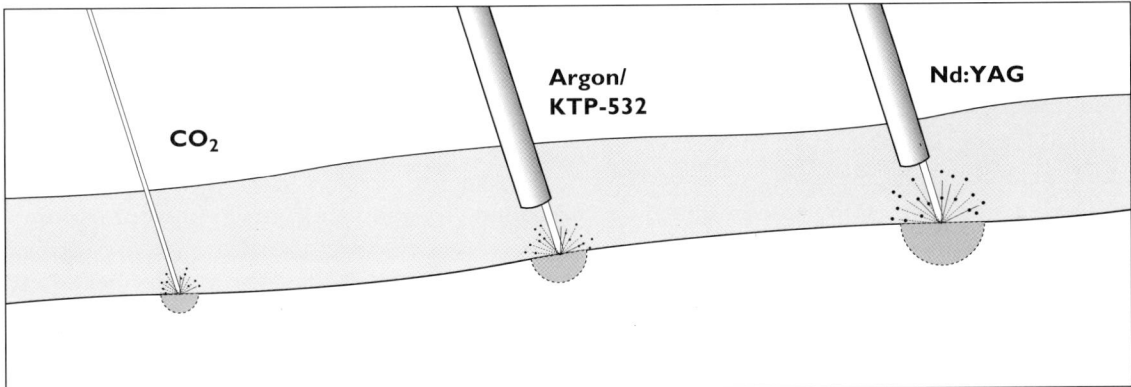

Figure 9.2 Schematic diagram comparing the depth of coagulative penetration and amount of scatter produced by various lasers

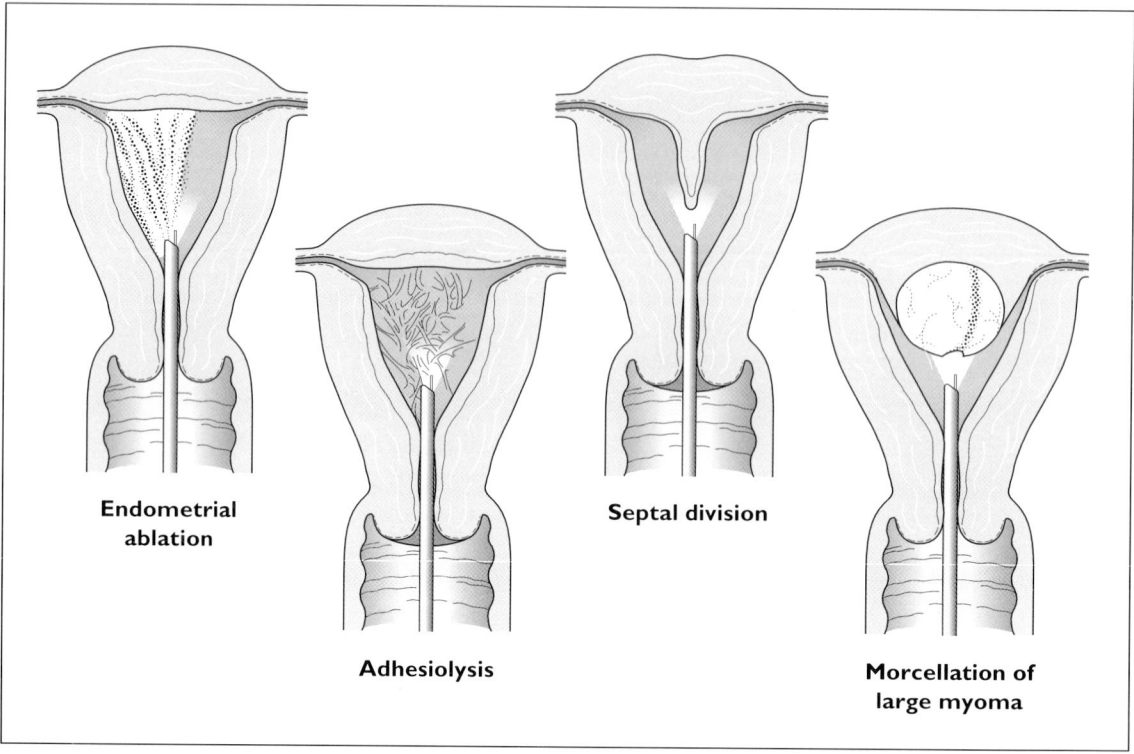

Endometrial ablation

Adhesiolysis

Septal division

Morcellation of large myoma

Figure 9.3 The most frequently performed hysteroscopic procedures performed with the use of fiberoptic lasers

for deep coagulation (4–5 mm), anterolateral scattering and penetration through fluids (Figure 9.4). Although bare fibers can be used to perform endometrial ablation, such fibers cannot be used for the more delicate operations that require controlled dissection and minimal tissue destruction, particularly peripherally, due to scattering. During removal of pedunculated leiomyomas, the bare fiber can be used to transect the pedicle flush to the uterine wall. In addition, morcellation of large fundal myomas can be accomplished using the same technique and, occasionally, myolysis of intramural myomatous tissue can be performed with sharp sculpted fibers that can penetrate this tissue.

As regards the treatment of polyps, an important aspect is their diagnosis. Treatment consists of blind removal of the polyp once the location has been determined,

using hysteroscopic scissors or a laser for pedunculated polyps, or a resectoscope for sessile polyps. However, a laser is an expensive tool for removal of a simple polyp.

To control and concentrate the laser beam at the tip of the fiber, these fibers are manufactured in different shapes, with sharp conical tips for precise cutting and ball-shaped tips for coagulation. These lasers do not need coaxial channels for cooling, unlike the sapphire tips that are attached to the laser fiber by metallic ferrules and require continuous cooling by gases or fluids to prevent melting. However, the use of CO_2 gas to cool the sapphire tip may result in fatal gas embolism due to the high rate of flow (500–1000 mL / min) required for effective cooling. Sapphire tips should never be used in the uterine cavity, not even with cooling fluids that will mix with the distending medium, thereby increasing the intrauterine pressure and predisposing the patient to fluid overload.

Although lasers can be used to treat other conditions such as uterine septa, intrauterine adhesions and uterine polyps, their use is somewhat restricted. Polyps do not require laser treatment and the cost involved greatly outweighs the benefit. Uterine septa, particularly broad septa, can be divided with sculpted sharp lasers that reduce both peripheral scattering and damage to the surrounding healthy endometrium. However, this type of energy should be used with the same precautions as when dividing septa with electrosurgery using the resectoscope. The cutting and coagulating power of the laser avoids bleeding, but does not permit observation of the small arterioles that may bleed upon reaching the myometrium. Therefore, special care should be taken to avoid inadvertent penetration of the myometrial wall.

Intrauterine adhesions can also be treated, using a sharp sculpted fiber for selective division of these adhesions. However, the possibility of scatter damage to the already compromised endometrium should always be considered and only sharp sculpted fibers should be used, as required. When using lasers to treat intrauterine adhesions, particularly those located laterally at the uterotubal cornua and lateral walls, a flexible operative hysteroscope is advantageous as the laser beam can be directed perpendicularly, permitting direct and precise targeting of the laser at the areas in need of treatment. This can be more difficult when rigid endoscopes are used to manipulate these lasers.

When using lasers for operative procedures, the fluids used to distend the uterus should contain electrolytes. Because such procedures may take an extended period of time, it is important to keep an accurate account of the amount of fluid used for distention and the amount recovered to determine the deficit of unrecovered fluid. Should the amount of unrecovered fluid exceed 1500 mL, particularly if the patient has a decreased urine output, diuretics can be administered which, in conjunction with close monitoring by the anesthesiologist, should prevent fluid overload.

Practical considerations in the use of lasers

Of the various fiberoptic lasers available, the coaxial type and those requiring continuous cooling, particularly with attached sapphire

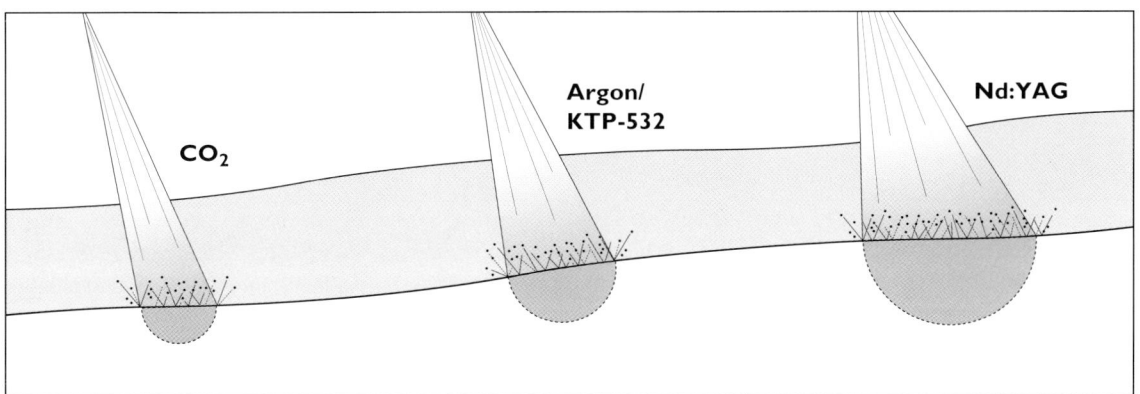

Figure 9.4 Schematic diagram showing the depth of coagulative penetration of tissue through fluid of the Nd:YAG laser compared with other lasers

tips as used in gastroenterology and / or orthopedic surgery, should not be used in the uterine cavity. The need for cooling by gases or fluids makes these lasers cumbersome to use and potentially dangerous. In particular, air, CO_2 or nitrogen to cool laser tips should never be used in the uterine cavity. Despite the coaxially injected fluids to cool sapphire tips, use of these lasers contributes to the intrauterine pressure and, thus, predisposes the patient to fluid overload by excessive absorption.

The lasers that can be used in gynecology are those with sculpted or extruded tips, whether sharp and conical for cutting or rounded for coagulation. These lasers permit a more precise application of the laser beam according to requirements and do not require continuous cooling. The appropriate fiber should be selected and the power required should also be displayed by the machine. The surgeon and the assisting personnel should be provided with protective glasses or goggles and the laser should be primed or activated in a 'tongue' blade with painted colored dots before being used on the patient. The activating pedal should be pressed only by the operator and not by the assistants, and only hysteroscopes with continuous-flow systems should be used to avoid excess fluid retention. The laser should be on a stand-by setting when not in use. It is important not to trip or bend the laser fibers excessively to avoid breakage. A special sign on the door of the operating suite should be displayed warning that a laser is in use and that persons entering the room require protective goggles. Only fluids containing electrolytes should be used with lasers, with meticulous monitoring of the amounts of fluid infused and recovered undertaken by the attending circulating nurse.

Selected bibliography

Baggish MS. A new laser hysteroscope for Nd-YAG endometrial ablation. *Lasers Surg Med* 1988;8:99

Baggish MS, Baltoyannis P. New techniques for laser ablation of the endometrium in high-risk patients. *Am J Obstet Gynecol* 1988; 159:287

Baggish MS, Daniell J. Death caused by air embolism associated with neodymium yttrium-alluminum-garnet laser surgery and artificial sapphire tips. *Am Obstet Gynecol* 1989;161:877

Baggish MS, Sze EHM, Morgan G. Hysteroscopic treatment of symptomatic submucous myomata uteri with the Nd-YAG laser. *J Gynecol Surg* 1989;5:27

Choe JK, Baggish MS. Hysteroscopic treatment of septate uterus with neodymium-YAG laser. *Fertil Steril* 1992;57:81

Daniell JF, Osher S, Miller W. Hysteroscopic resection of uterine septi with visible light laser energy. *Colpo Gynecol Laser Surg* 1987; 3:217

Diamond MP, Boyers SP, Lavy G, *et al.* Endoscopic use of the potassium-titanyl-phosphate 532 laser in gynecologic surgery. *Colpo Gynecol Laser Surg* 1987;3:213

Goldrath MH, Fuller T, Segal S. Laser photovaporization of endometrium for the treatment of menorrhagia. *Am J Obstet Gynecol* 1981;140:14

Newton RJ, Mackenzie WE, Emens MJ, Jordan JA. Division of uterine adhesions (Asherman's syndrome) with the Nd-YAG laser. *Br J Obstet Gynaecol* 1989;96:102

10 Hormonal preparation of the endometrium

The performance of hysteroscopy, particularly operative hysteroscopy, is usually timed to take place during the early follicular phase once menstruation has ceased in premenopausal patients. This is to avoid the thick luxurious endometrium encountered following ovulation (Figures 10.1 and 10.2). When the endometrium is thin and regular, hysteroscopic examination is greatly facilitated. Surgery can be accomplished without unnecessary obscuring of the view by debris, mucus or tissue floating in the distending medium. While such timing is sufficient for most hysteroscopic procedures, there are two specific procedures that require additional hormonal treatment to prepare these patients for surgery, namely, endometrial ablation and (occasionally) submucous myomectomy.

During endometrial ablation, particularly when laser or electrosurgical coagulation is to be used, it is important that the endometrium be as thin (1–2 mm) and uniform as possible. This is necessary to permit the beam to penetrate and destroy

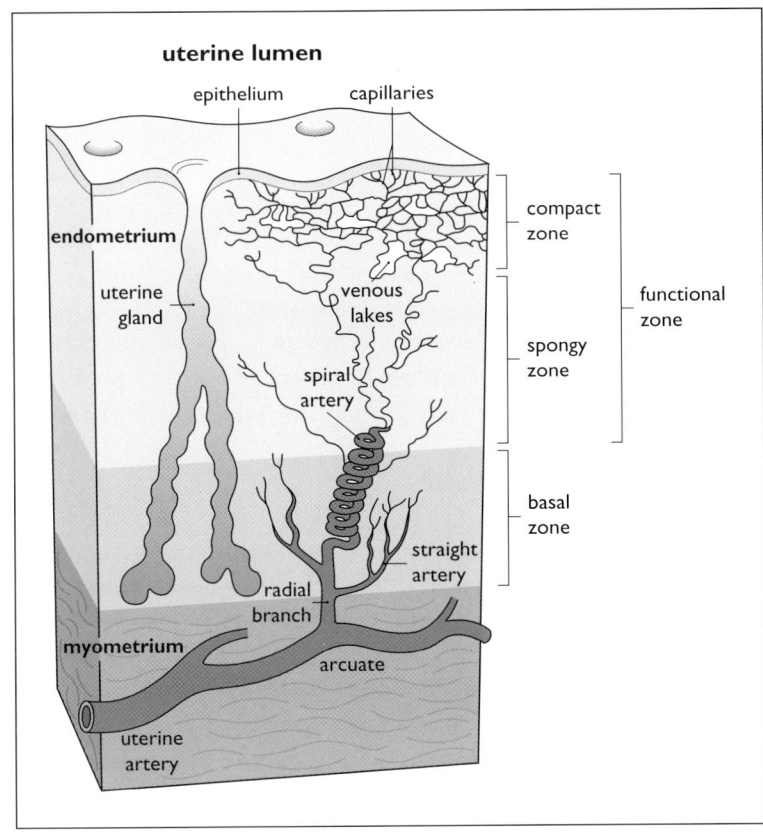

Figure 10.1 Schematic diagram of the development of normal endometrium

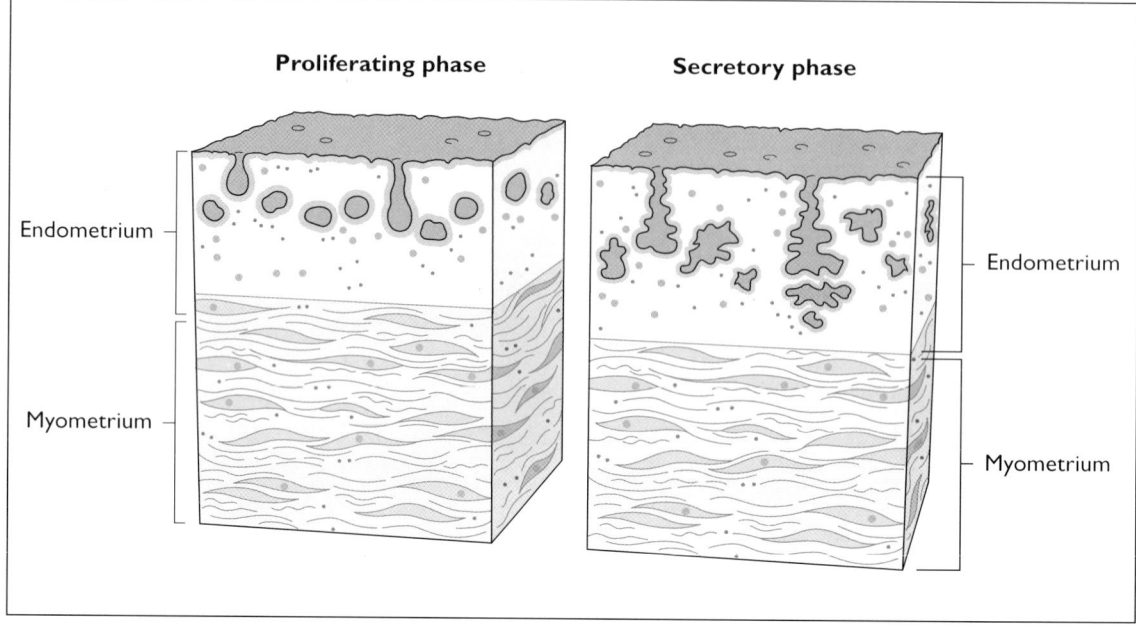

Figure 10.2 Schematic diagram showing changes in the endometrium during the proliferative and secretory phases of the menstrual cycle

not only the endometrium, including the basal layer, but also the superficial (2–3 mm) portion of the myometrium to avoid recurrences. This effect can best be obtained by treating the endometrium hormonally prior to surgery.

Several pharmacological agents cause thinning and atrophy of the endometrium, including progesterone, danazol and Gn-RH analogues. In the absence of these agents, both mechanical and suction curettage have been used to remove the functional endometrial lining prior to endometrial ablation.

Progesterone

Endometrial thinning and atrophy can be achieved with high doses of medroxyprogesterone acetate (Provera®), 20–30 mg / day, for 4–6 weeks. Weekly injections of either hydrosoluble progesterone 100 mg or megestrol acetate (Megace®) 20–30 mg / day can also be given for 6 weeks. Whereas the depot forms of medroxyprogesterone acetate have

been used with one–two shots 4–6 weeks apart, the results are rather unpredictable as reabsorption cannot be controlled. Although progesterones induce endometrial atrophy, they usually achieve this goal over a long period of time and high doses are necessary. Within only 4–6 weeks, there is a paradoxical response of cell decidualization, resulting in an endometrium that is thicker and more irregular and may hamper visualization. Furthermore, the side effects of these medications, such as depression and water retention, may result in poor patient compliance.

Danazol

Danazol can achieve endometrial atrophy with 800 mg / day orally for 6 weeks. The endometrium is markedly decreased and, although the endometrial atrophy is more uniform and consistent than that with the progesterones, some patients may not be able to tolerate the secondary androgenic side effects.

Gonadotropin-releasing hormone (Gn-RH) analogues

The advent of continuous-use Gn-RH analogues, particularly those in depot form, has facilitated hormonal preparation of the endometrium as these compounds produce a profound hypoestrogenic state and, subsequently, uniform atrophy of the endometrium. However, because they are agonists, there is usually a flare-up phase of 2–3 weeks before the desensitization phase, with a drop in gonadotropins. Although administration during the late luteal phase somewhat blunts the agonistic phase, the initial flare-up still occurs in most patients. When using depot forms such as depot Lupron 3.75 mg intramuscularly, endometrial ablation can be performed a month later. However, a significant number of patients will not achieve complete atrophy of the endometrium within this time due to the variability of the flare-up phase which may result in only 1–2 weeks of desensitization, which may not be sufficient for endometrial atrophy. Approximately 25–30% of patients may still have thickened endometrium following desensitization. For this reason, it is useful to give a second injection 4 weeks after the first to ensure complete and sufficient desensitization, and which may produce an atrophic endometrium in more than 95% of these patients (Figure 10.3).

Although most patients require a 3.75-mg intramuscular injection, some patients with marked obesity may benefit more from a 7.5-mg dose. Endometrial ablation is then

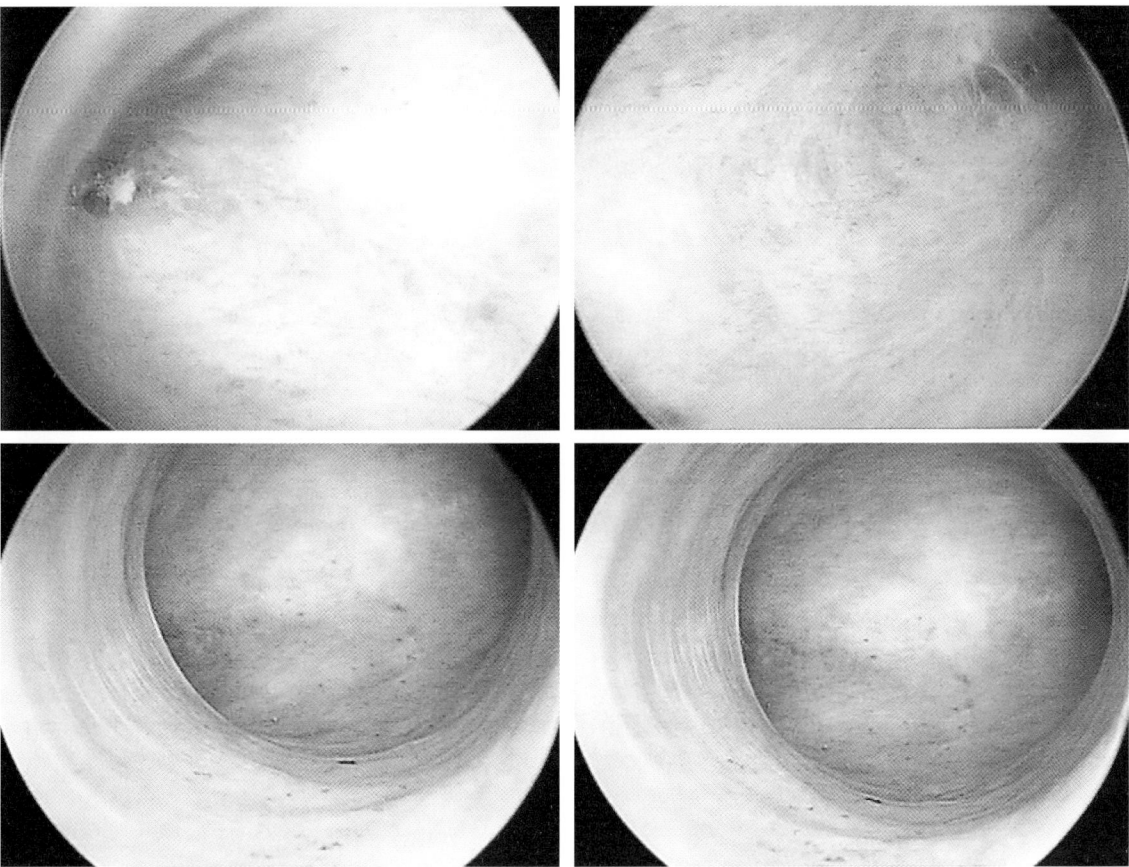

Figure 10.3 Hysteroscopic views of atrophic endometrium

scheduled to take place 2–3 weeks following the second injection.

Hormonal preparation of the endometrium is also useful in patients with submucous leiomyomas before they undergo resectoscopic or hysteroscopic myomectomy. The endometrium becomes thinner, permitting better visualization during myomectomy. Should patients bleed excessively, which is usually the case with these types of myomas, the procedure can be performed after the bleeding is controlled. This is particularly useful if the patient is anemic as it reestablishes normal levels of hemoglobin and permits, if necessary, storage of autologous blood. The use of Gn-RH analogues, which are now the preferred method for preparing these patients for surgery, provides additional benefits to facilitate myomectomy: decreased vascularization due to a reduced blood flow; some reduction in the size of the leiomyoma, which makes the procedure easier to perform; and a more predictable cessation of abnormal bleeding. In general, depot Lupron at 3.75 mg intramuscularly is administered in three doses as monthly injections. The decision whether to use adjuncts or not is based on the individual patient, taking into account the bleeding, hemoglobin levels, and size and type of leiomyoma as those with an intramural component almost always require this type of preparation.

Other hysteroscopic therapeutic procedures that require good visualization of the uterine cavity, an absence of debris and a thin endometrium include division of uterine septa and tubal cannulation. In these cases, if the procedures are performed in the immediate postmenstrual period, hormonal preparation is usually not necessary. Those patients who bleed abnormally because of oligoovulation may benefit from hormonal preparation of the endometrium.

Other adjuncts to hysteroscopic surgery

Prophylactic antibiotics

Prophylactic antibiotics are used routinely in the treatment of uterine septa. They are usually administered by intravenous injection during the operation with 3–4 days of oral maintenance treatment. Patients treated for intrauterine adhesions are also given prophylactic antibiotics preoperatively and 3–4 days postoperatively as maintenance treatment if an intrauterine splint is not used. When intrauterine splints are used, the therapy is continued for 7 days orally.

Tubal cannulation may also require prophylactic antibiotics intraoperatively. The regimens vary, but the most commonly used antibiotics are the cephalosporins such as cephazolin or similar, 1 g intravenously 'piggyback' during the operation, followed by 500 mg of cephalexin orally four times a day. Alternatively, doxycycline 100 mg intravenously is used during the operation, piggybacked, followed by 100 mg twice daily orally for 4 days.

Estrogen and progesterone treatment

Estrogens in the form of conjugated estrogens (Premarin®) are given in doses of 2.5 mg twice daily for 30 days after division of uterine septa, followed by medroxyprogesterone acetate 10 mg / day orally during the last 7 days of the cycle to ensure withdrawal bleeding. Patients with moderate-to-severe intrauterine adhesions are also prescribed this estrogen regimen for 30–40 days. Although there is no evidence that these regimens are better than no treatment, on an empirical basis and by ultrasound measurements, they appear to expedite endometrial growth.

Hormonal preparation

For endometrial ablation, the following regimens are useful: danazol 800 mg / day in four doses for 6 weeks; depot Lupron 3.75 mg intramuscularly in two doses 1 month apart, except for patients who weigh more than 250 pounds (114 kg), in which case the dose is increased to 7.5 mg intramuscularly.

Myomas are also treated, if bleeding is excessive and continuous, the patient is anemic or the myoma is >3 cm, with depot Lupron 3.75 mg intramuscularly (in three doses) 1 month apart. In anemic patients, the treatment may be continued until the hemoglobin and hematocrit levels are normalized.

Hysterosalpingogram

Hysterosalpingography is performed, if the patient desires pregnancy, 3 months after myomectomy to ensure that the symmetry of the uterine cavity is reestablished. Following removal of intrauterine adhesions, hysterosalpingography can be performed after the hormonal treatment, particularly in moderate-to-severe cases, to ascertain normalcy of the uterine cavity and tubal patency. After division of a uterine septum and once hormonal treatment has been completed, a hysterosalpingogram should be obtained following menstruation to assess the symmetry of the uterine cavity. After tubal cannulation, a hysterosalpingogram is mandatory if pregnancy does not occur within 1 year.

Ultrasonography

Vaginal sonography is used preoperatively when leiomyomas are present, and postoperatively if the leiomyoma is partially intramural and not totally resected. Vaginal sonography should be performed to assess the status of the remaining partially treated leiomyoma 3–6 months following the procedure, or earlier if the patient becomes symptomatic. Fluid-enhanced sonography may also be carried out if the information obtained by vaginal sonography alone remains inadequate.

Selected bibliography

Brooks PG, Serden SP, Davos I. Hormonal inhibition of the endometrium for resectoscopic endometrial ablation. *Am J Obstet Gynecol* 1991;164:1601

Droegemueller N, Herbst AL, Mishell DR, Stenchever MA. Abnormal uterine bleeding. In *Comprehensive Gynecology*. St Louis: CV Mosby, 1987:953–64

Goldrath MH. Use of danazol in hysteroscopic surgery for menorrhagia. *J Reprod Med* 1990;35:91

Ke RW, Taylor PJ. Endometrial ablation to control excessive uterine bleeding. *Hum Reprod* 1991;6:574

Perino A, Chianchiano N, Petronio M, *et al.* Role of leuprolide acetate depot in hysteroscopic surgery: A controlled study. *Fertil Steril* 1993;59:507

Rich AD, Manyonda IT, Patel R, Amias AG. A comparison of the efficacy of danazol, norethisterone, cyproterone acetate and medroxyprogesterone acetate in endometrial thinning prior to ablation: A pilot study. *Gynaecol Endosc* 1995;4:59

Valle RF. Endometrial ablation for dysfunctional uterine bleeding: Role of Gn-RH agonists. *Int J Gynecol Obstet* 1993;41:3

Valle RF. Assessing new treatments for dysfunctional uterine bleeding. *Contemp Obstet Gynecol* 1994;4:43

11 Video hysteroscopy and documentation

Diagnostic and therapeutic hysteroscopic procedures should be documented with diagrams, particularly in those cases that require operative intervention. It is important to outline and depict the findings and treatment in the diagram, particularly for those procedures that require follow-up and which may require additional procedures in the future. Simple drawings are useful as a complement to the operative report (Figure 11.1).

Still pictures

While still pictures were used more extensively in the 1970s and 1980s as part of the documentation, with the advent of video, this valuable means of documentation has become somewhat neglected. Nevertheless, still photographs remain the best and simplest method of documenting important findings and important steps in an operative procedure. In addition, pictures in the form of 35-mm transparencies are useful for educational purposes.

Video systems

Video has become an integral part of endoscopy particularly because of its improved resolution and versatility. Small videocameras are easily adapted for attachment to the ocular parts of the hysteroscope or resectoscope, and operations can be performed under video monitoring. Video hysteroscopy was difficult before the new high-sensitivity cameras were introduced

particularly because of the need to provide powerful light sources to enable photography of the hysteroscopic procedures. At present, most cameras can be used through small endoscopes during diagnostic and operative procedures. Special cameras that are highly light-sensitive have been introduced specifically for this purpose (Figure 11.2). During operative procedures with a hysteroscope, the wide-angle view and high resolution of such a camera facilitates the performance of the procedure and confers greater accuracy when treating specific conditions. Similarly, when the resectoscope is used, the videocamera permits a clearer view of the field and tissues, which is particularly important when dissecting, cutting or removing lesions (Figure 11.3). Video has also made it easier to assess different tissues, thereby rendering electrosurgery safer. In addition, the surgeon is able to operate in a comfortable position that does not require major effort, as is the case when the operator must keep his eye to the hysteroscopic ocular during operations with endoscopes. Finally, the procedure is shared with the operating team, thus increasing interest, and enhancing their participation and help.

The new video printers and digital photographic units have greatly facilitated the production of video prints and slides with excellent color reproduction. Thus, there is no longer the necessity to interrupt both the videorecording of the operation and the operation itself to take a still photograph. Digital photography units can

PRENTICE WOMEN'S HOSPITAL AND MATERNITY CENTER
OF
NORTHWESTERN MEMORIAL HOSPITAL

REPORT OF HYSTEROSCOPIC EXAMINATION

NAME _____ HOSPITAL NO. _____ DATE _____
AGE _____ PARITY _____ LAST PREGNANCY _____ LMP _____
METHOD OF CONTRACEPTION _____ CLINICAL HISTORY_____
_____
PREOPERATIVE DIAGNOSIS _____
EXAMINATION: 1ST _____ REPEAT _____
SURGEON _____ ASSISTANT _____
ANESTHESIA: GENERAL _____ LOCAL _____ ANALGESIA _____
UTERINE DISTENTION: MEDIUM _____ QUANTITY_____
ADEQUATE _____ INADEQUATE _____
QUALITY OF VISUALIZATION: SATISFACTORY _____ UNSATISFACTORY _____
FINDINGS _____
HYSTEROSCOPIC OPERATION _____

DIAGRAM

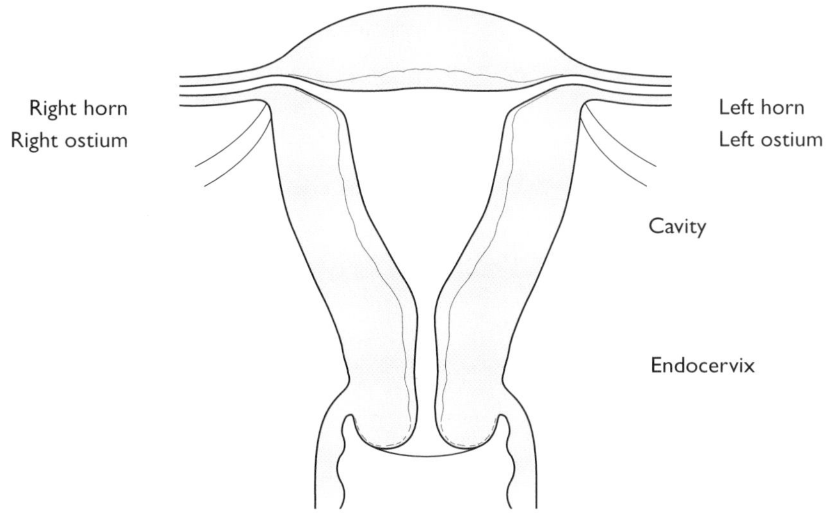

Right horn
Right ostium

Left horn
Left ostium

Cavity

Endocervix

DX _____
ANCILLARY PROCEDURE _____
COMPLICATIONS _____
INTRAUTERINE PHOTOGRAPHS: ❏ YES ❏ NO
_____ M.D.

Figure 11.1 Sample report for documenting hysteroscopic examination findings

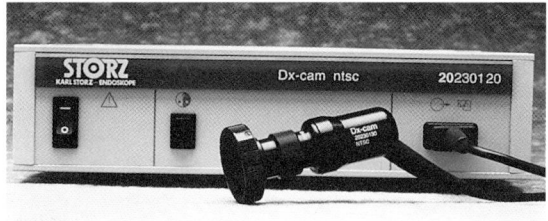

Figure 11.2 Highly light-sensitive camera specially designed for endoscopic procedures

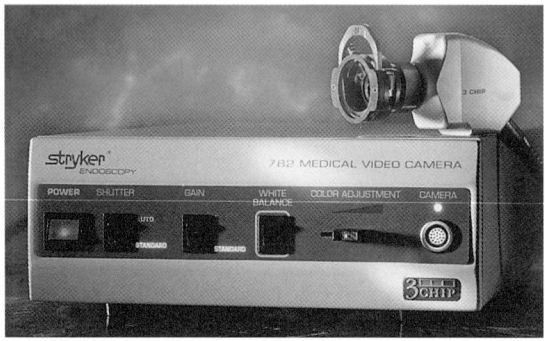

Figure 11.3 A 3-chip videocamera for endoscopy

provide this type of documentation instantaneously; either the operator or an assistant can activate the unit at will whenever a photograph is required. This type of technology has become standard in most operating suites equipped with endoscopic systems.

Practical points for video

It is important to prepare for videotaping before the procedure begins. The machine should be checked, a clean tape inserted and the machine activated. Should a video print function be available, the pedal to obtain such pictures should be placed close to the operator. Before introduction into the patient, the camera should be connected to the hysteroscope and / or resectoscope, the colors made uniform and the focusing completed. Moisture should be prevented from entering the ocular and camera lenses. If this occurs, the lenses should be cleaned with a soft dry cloth. The colors and brightness of the camera should be adapted as necessary, using conventional or standard light-sensitive cameras or a special camera with even greater sensitivity to light. The light source can be increased or decreased, according to requirements.

Selected bibliography

Acland RD. Photomicrography through the operating microscope. *Plastic Reconstruct Surg* 1977;60:730

Brooks PG. Video endoscopy cameras and printers to assist surgeons. *Contemp OB / GYN. Technology* 1989;43–7

Kent PR, Malinak R. Intraoperative photography. A sterile system. *Obstet Gynecol* 1978;52:365

Marlow J. Endoscopic photography. In Baggish MS, ed. *Gynecologic Endoscopy and Instrumentation. Clinical Obstetrics and Gynecology.* Hagerstown, MD: Harper & Row, 1983:359–65

Marlow JL. Hysteroscopic photography. In Baggish MS, Barbot J, Valle RF, eds. *Diagnostic and Operative Hysteroscopy. A Text and Atlas.* Chicago: Year Book Medical Publishers, 1989:215–22

12 Learning hysteroscopy and resectoscopy for credentialing

The learning process for any surgical procedure should begin with recognition of the normal anatomy and its abnormal variations. Therefore, diagnostic hysteroscopy should always be the first step in the learning curve.

There are several methods available today for learning diagnostic hysteroscopy. Inanimate models are most useful for testing the instruments and their direction of view – specifically, foreoblique vision – and the movements necessary for a general inspection. After inanimate models, the transition to animal models is easier; different distending media can be used and the mechanisms involved in working the various systems explored. Cow uteri and pig bladders are easily obtainable and can be mounted on small platforms; extirpated uteri after hysterectomy can also be used as models for learning the fundamentals of this type of endoscopy (Figure 12.1).

Once the instrumentation, different distending media and techniques have become familiar, the physician can perform

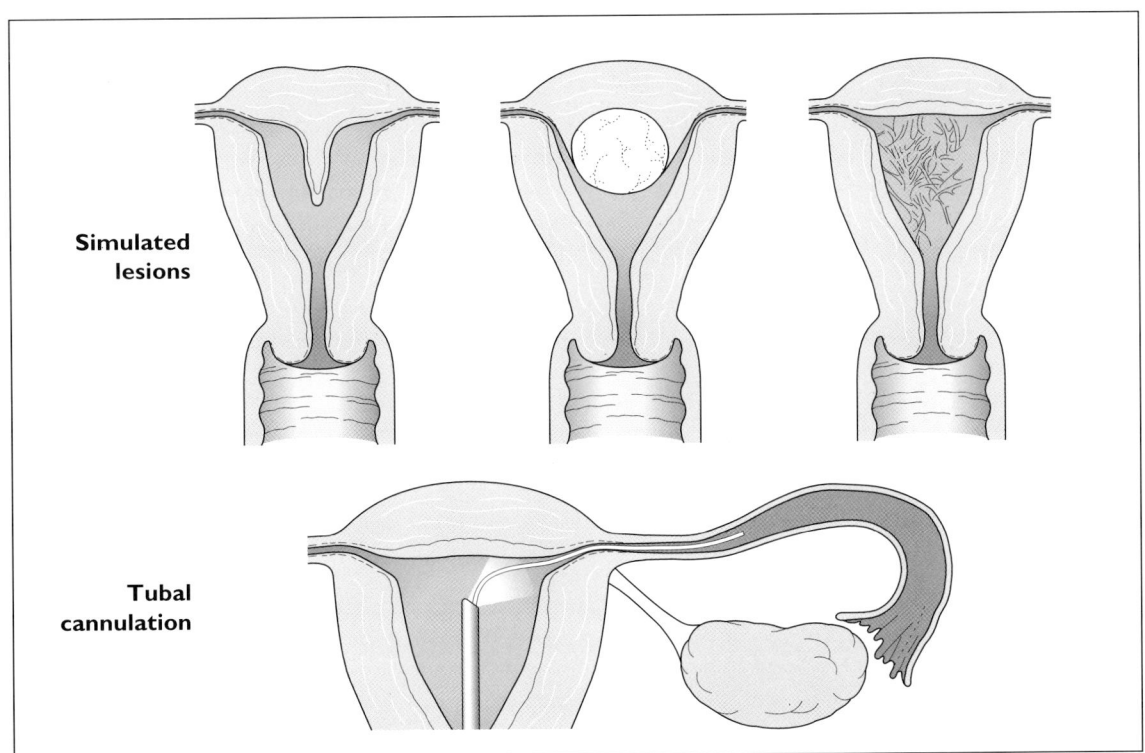

Simulated lesions

Tubal cannulation

Figure 12.1 Different exercises for practicing procedures using extirpated uteri and simulated lesions

the procedures in live patients in the operating room. It is useful to begin with a patient who is under general anesthesia, as this permits the use of the instruments without undue hesitation, thereby allowing more time for examination and dealing with any problems that may arise with the instrumentation; the operator is also free of any worry of being observed by the patient. In general, patients who require curettage for evaluation of abnormal bleeding are excellent candidates. Before attempting the clinical application of these procedures, hysteroscopy should be performed in patients who have no pathology such as those who require tubal sterilization, or in patients prior to a vaginal hysterectomy.

The use of hysteroscopy therapeutically should only be attempted after having mastered the diagnostic techniques, as the therapeutic procedures require greater experience with the instruments. Inanimate models may be useful, such as plastic uterine models with pathological lesions that can be dissected and removed. Green peppers or melons can be used to simulate the uterus (Figure 12.2); different structures and multiple seeds can be grasped with grasping or rigid forceps. Bands of tissue can be cut to simulate division of a septum or an adhesion. Cardboard boxes can be constructed into different obstacles that will serve as lesions to be removed or divided. The physician can then move on to animal models, such as cow uteri or pig bladders containing simulated pathological lesions, such as tissue sutured to the walls to simulate polyps or myomas, sutures in the midline to simulate a septum, or sutures from wall to wall at different places to simulate adhesions. These exercises help to acquire dexterity in the manipulation of semirigid or flexible instruments through the hysteroscopic operating channel. Furthermore, while operating, the direction of view can be changed from one place to another and the physician can observe the changes that occur within the simulated cavity and correlate them later to observations during an actual operation.

The use of the resectoscope also requires special instruction. The instrument should be well known in all its components, and assembled and disassembled to gain an understanding of how the various parts fit together in the system. The most often performed procedures with a resectoscope

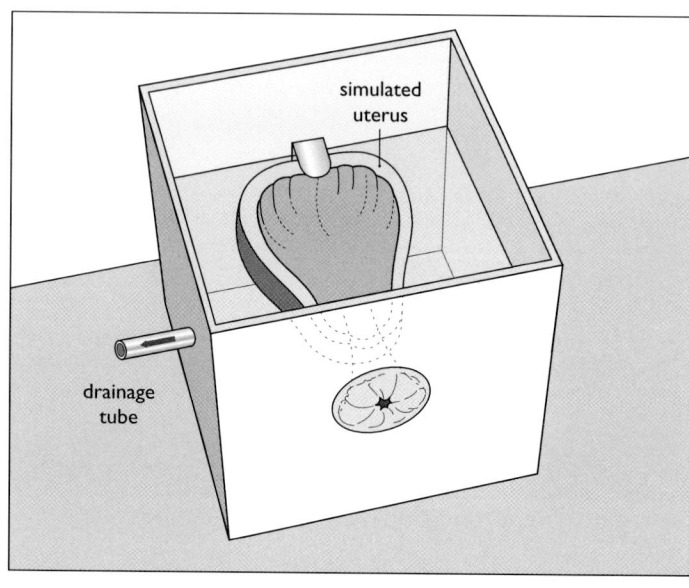

Figure 12.2 Model boxes devised for training use various materials to simulate lesions and anatomical structures

can be attempted on surfaces such as a raw potato to simulate myomas that can be resected with a loop while embedded in a non-electrolyte-containing fluid. Before the resectoscope is activated, special grounding of all these substances is necessary. Liver or other similar tissues can also be coagulated and resected under simulated circumstances. The transition is then made to extirpated pig bladders or cow uteri with different lesions attached, representing various pathological conditions to be resected and / or coagulated. The roller-ball / bar electrodes can be used to simulate endometrial ablation by coagulation in these specimens to demonstrate how these instruments are activated and rolled, and what their effect on tissues is.

Physicians who want to learn how to use fiberoptic lasers should use the operative hysteroscope with activated lasers on specimens simulating the human uterus. A bare fiber and both the contact or dragging technique and the non-contact blanching technique for coagulation should be used to learn their different effects on tissue. The same precautions (special goggles or filters) as those taken in the operating suite should be exercised when these lasers are used and activated to protect the eyes from retinal injury.

Anesthesia

At the beginning of the learning curve, most procedures, whether diagnostic or therapeutic, but particularly the latter, should be performed under general anesthesia. Once experience and confidence are acquired, diagnostic procedures can be attempted under local anesthesia. This is important not only to avoid frustration but, if the procedure does not go as planned, to prevent undue concern by the patient. Regional anesthesia is appropriate for most hysteroscopic and / or resectoscopic procedures unless laparoscopy is planned. Nevertheless, the patient's wishes should be respected as many will only accept general anesthesia. If cervical dilatation is required while using local anesthesia and the dilatation is difficult or the patient becomes uncomfortable, it is preferable to abort the procedure and change the anesthetic to make the patient comfortable. If local anesthesia fails to produce its effect and the operator persists in attempting to complete the cervical dilatation, the result may be more anxiety and a painful experience for the patient. Therefore, these patients require other anesthetics at different settings.

Preceptorships

Although diagnostic and operative hysteroscopy can be learned by reading, observing and reviewing photographs and videos, the availability of a preceptor is important. A preceptor can encourage progress, correct mistakes, expedite the learning curve and guide the practitioner in performing the procedure more safely. Preceptorships are most useful when operative procedures are to be learned, whether with a hysteroscope or resectoscope. A preceptor can help not only in the performance of a procedure itself, but also in setting the system up to be particularly effective for learning the procedure and in helping the assisting team, especially the nurses, to establish a standard arrangement for the instruments and any additional requirements, such as delivery of the distending media, placement of the video system and monitoring of electrical or laser energies. In addition, the preceptor can attest to the ability of the practitioner to perform specific procedures safely once the preceptorship is completed.

It is important, having learned the hysteroscopic / resectoscopic procedures, to maintain proficiency, as with any other surgical procedure.

All therapeutic hysteroscopic procedures require knowledge of diagnostic hysteroscopy. All practitioners must show evidence of having: attended a formal course on indications, contraindications and possible complications; attended a laboratory workshop designed to teach how to perform these procedures; knowledge of physics and the basic principles of electrosurgery as well as laser energies; and appropriate credentialing in the performance of minor and major gynecological procedures.

Selected bibliography

American College of Gynecologists and Obstetricians. *Credentialing Guidelines for New Operative Procedures, ACGO Committee Opinion, No. 142.* Washington, DC: ACGO, 1994

American College of Surgeons. Statement of emerging surgical technologies and the evaluation of credentials. *Am Coll Surg Bull* 1994;79:40

Barak G. The learning curve (Editorial). *J Am Med Assoc* 1993;270:1280

Cass OW, Freeman ML, Peine CJ, *et al.* Objective evaluation of endoscopy skills during training. *Ann Intern Med* 1993;118:40

Gimpelson RJ, Schomburg ME, Bagby ML. An animal model for learning Nd:YAG laser ablation of the endometrium. *J Reprod Med* 1989;39:461

Hatlie MJ. Climbing 'the learning curve'. New technologies, emerging obligations. *J Am Med Assoc* 1989;270:1364

Keye WR. Hitting a moving target: Credentialing the endoscopic surgeon. *Fertil Steril* 1994; 62:1115

Sanmarco MJ, Youngblood JP. A resident teaching program in operative endoscopy. *Obstet Gynecol* 1993;81:463

Siegler AM. Learning and teaching hysteroscopic tubal sterilization. In Sciarra JJ, Butler JC, Speidel JJ, eds. *Hysteroscopic Sterilization.* New York: Intercontinental Medical Book Corporation, 1974:113–43

Society for Reproductive Surgeons and The American Fertility Society. Guidelines for attaining privileges in gynecologic operative endoscopy. *Fertil Steril* 1994;62:1118

Tulandi T. Canadian guidelines for training in operative endoscopy (Letter to the Editor). *Gynaecol Endosc* 1995;4:69

Wolfe WM, Levine RL, Sanfilippo JS, Eggler S. A teaching model for endoscopic surgery: Hysteroscopy and pelviscopy surgery. *Fertil Steril* 1988;50:662

13 Hysterosalpingography and laparoscopy in infertility

Alvin M. Siegler

Hysterosalpingography (HSG) in the 1990s remains an important screening procedure during an investigation of infertility despite a number of limitations: the radiological examination cannot detect endometriosis or significant pelvic adhesions. It has been estimated that approximately 300 000 diagnostic hysterosalpingograms are performed in the USA annually and the format has not changed in decades. Indeed, most studies are still carried out with spot films without fluoroscopy[1]. Around one-third of these examinations are performed by radiologists alone and another third by gynecologists alone; in the remainder of cases, both groups of physicians are involved in the procedure. In a recent survey of hospitals in Liverpool in the UK, the authors reported that around 100 HSGs are performed each year in the hospitals surveyed[2].

Technique

HSG is performed in the preovulatory phase as an outpatient procedure. Less than 20% of women require sedation and antispasmodic agents. Patients with a history of pelvic inflammatory disease or a positive culture for *Chlamydia* or gonorrhea should be given antibacterial prophylaxis. Water-soluble contrast material is either injected through a metal cannula or a Foley catheter balloon. An HSG study usually requires 4–5 spot films to be taken under fluoroscopic image intensification using 6–8 mL of contrast material, the amount depending on the size of the uterine cavity (Figure 13.1)[3].

Proximal tubal obstruction is suspected if the cornua are pointed rather than rounded, with absence of tubal filling after contrast material has been injected. Tubal filling with spill and spread of the contrast material on the drainage film indicates tubal patency, although the proximal segment should always be examined for tubal polyps or diverticula.

Technical variations include the use of 70 mm and 105 mm radiographs, technetium-99 HSG as an alternative to contrast HSG[4] cinefluoroscopy, low-dose scanning-beam digital HSG, radionuclide studies to assess tubal patency[5] and, recently, an attempt to

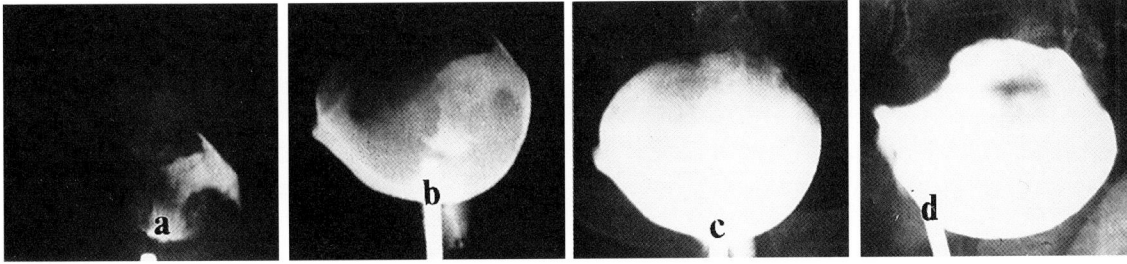

Figure 13.1 This enlarged uterine cavity (**d**) was due to a submucous myoma. Fractional instillation of contrast material (**a–c**) outlines the cavity and reveals the defect

correlate tubal perfusion pressures and opacification by standardizing the injection volume per time intervals[6].

Errors in technique (Figure 13.2) and interpretation of HSGs are frequently a cause for discrepancies when the results are compared with the findings at laparoscopy. The most common reason for failure to visualize the uterine cavity is inadequate traction on the cervix or obstruction of the view of the lower uterine segment because of either the catheter bulb or an opaque speculum[7]. As failure to opacify tubes can be due to the use of inadequate amounts of contrast material, the endpoint of stopping the contrast injection is either an increase in lower abdominal pain or evidence of vascular intravasation. Failure to obtain a drainage film will prevent adequate evaluation of the filled tube and miss the diagnosis of fimbrial phimosis. The delayed film helps to differentiate distal tubal obstruction from tubal patency.

Tubes are considered normal if bilateral tubal fill-and-spill is seen with normal rugae markings and without localization on the drainage film (Figure 13.3). The isthmic segment should show a thin linear opacification. An abnormal salpingogram is defined as the presence of distal tubal occlusion with or without a hydrosalpinx. A salpingogram

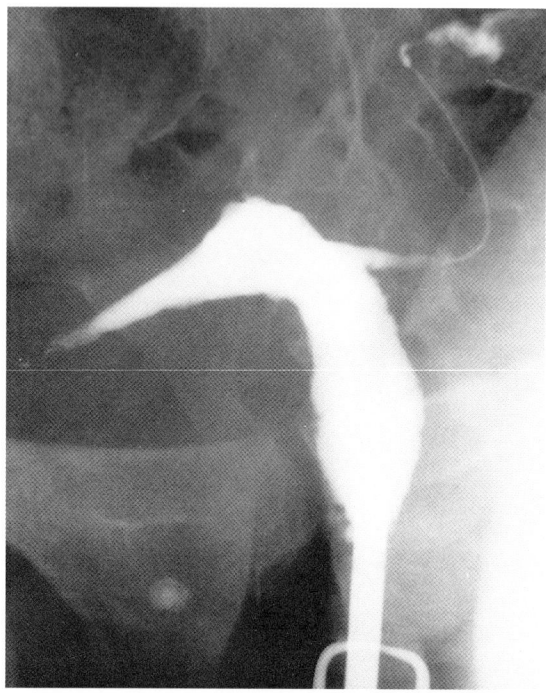

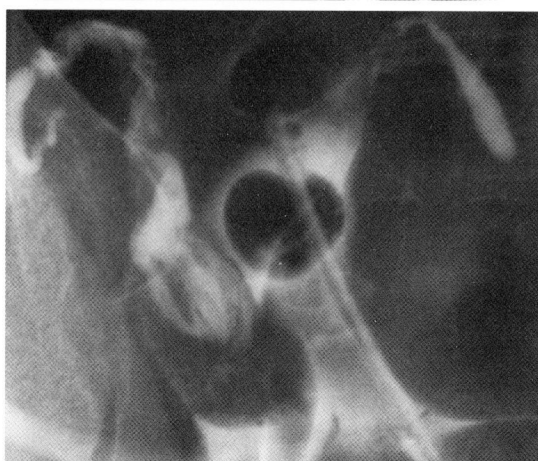

Figure 13.2 A common technical error in hysterosalpingography is caused by failure to exert sufficient traction on the cervical tenaculum (upper). Tubes will fail to opacify if the balloon catheter is inserted too far into the uterine cavity (lower)

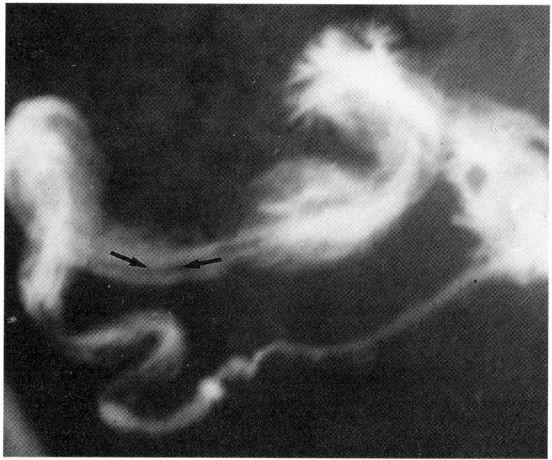

Figure 13.3 Normal appearances of the Fallopian tube on hysterosalpingography include clear rugal markings (arrows)

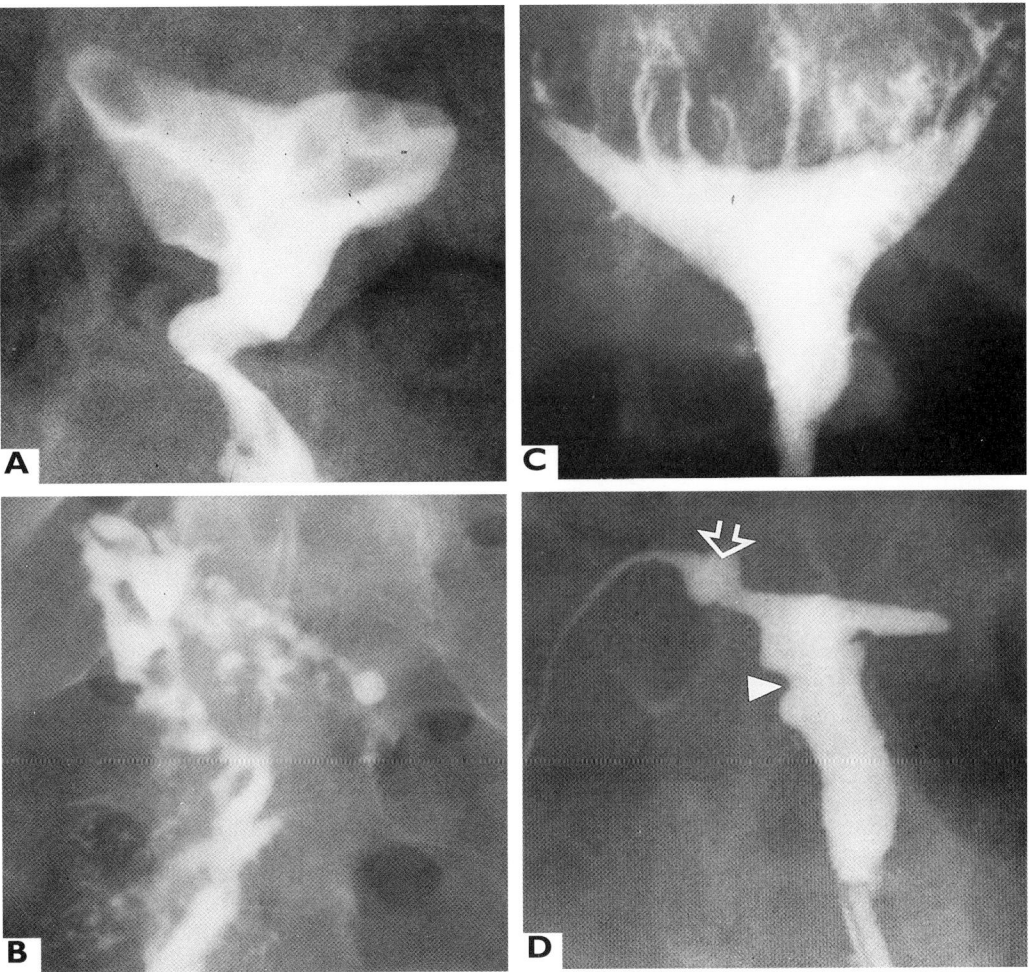

Figure 13.4 (**A**) These multiple intrauterine filling defects were due to endometrial polyps; (**B**) this case of severe intrauterine distortion was caused by advanced intrauterine adhesions; (**C**) this appearance of myometrial intravasation was due to adenomyosis; (**D**) the effects of diethylstilbestrol *in utero* include a tubal bulge (open arrow) and an intrauterine defect (solid arrow)

is considered suspicious or equivocal if there is partial tubal filling, or if proximal tubal obstruction is seen or different sites of occlusion are found in each tube.

An HSG that is adequately performed and carefully interpreted remains an excellent screening test for uterine and tubal abnormalities because of its ability to outline the lumina of the Fallopian tubes and uterine cavity. The radiological study should be able to detect congenital uterine abnormalities, intrauterine adhesions and submucosal tumors such as polyps or myomas (Figures 13.4 and 13.5).

Laparoscopy used for diagnosis can locate and stage endometriosis, classify the severity of periadnexal adhesions, examine the uterine serosal surface, and evaluate the size, consistency and patency of the Fallopian tubes. The endoscopic examination can study more precisely the fimbriated ends of the Fallopian tubes.

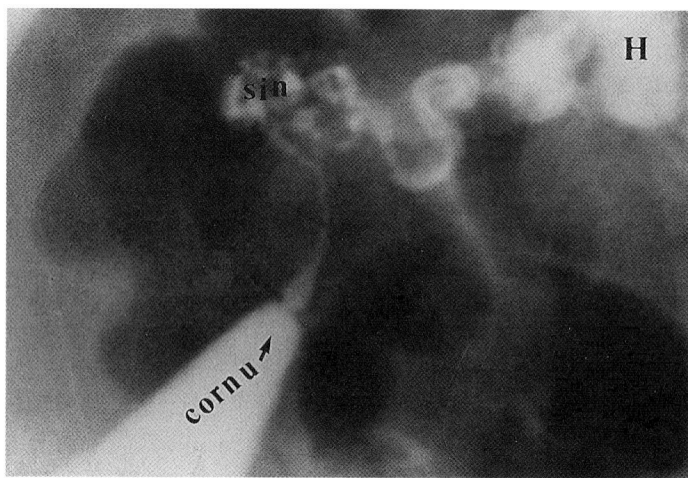

Figure 13.5 This Fallopian tube shows bipolar disease with salpingitis isthmica nodosa (sin) and hydrosalpinx (H)

Contrast material

What is the therapeutic effect of the HSG? Pregnancy rates following the use of oil-based (OBCM) and water-based contrast materials (WBCM) have been confounded by a number of variables. In an effort to compare the therapeutic effects of OBCM and WBCM, 29 patients who were found to have normal pelvic anatomy at laparoscopy were randomized to receive either OBCM ($n = 15$) or WBCM ($n = 14$). A significant difference in pregnancy rates was noted: 40% in those receiving OBCM and 14% in the WBCM group. These observations were confirmed in another study which showed significantly more term pregnancies with the use of an ethiodized poppyseed oil for HSG than with the use of three water-soluble contrast media groups[8,9]. A potential mechanism for fertility enhancement was suggested by a study which showed the ability of contrast material and / or indigo–carmine dye to inhibit lymphocytic proliferation and phagocytosis by macrophages in the peritoneal fluid[10].

Catheterization

Although the debate as regards selection of the best contrast material is still ongoing, one of the most significant additions to HSG has been the introduction of interventional and imaging techniques that offer new therapeutic possibilities[11–14]. The diagnosis of proximal tubal obstruction made by HSG and confirmed by laparoscopy is not invariably followed by tubocornual anastomosis because transcervical selective salpingography (TSS) is now available as the contemporary approach to non-opacification of the Fallopian tube. Fluoroscopically guided coaxial catheterization and canalization has resulted in tubal patency in so many cases that the procedure has become a prerequisite before attempting microsurgical anastomosis. However, in certain carefully selected patients, the data suggest that the more costly and more invasive endoscopic procedures are the best first choice as either diagnostic or therapeutic procedures. Such an approach requires renewed cooperation between the gynecologist and radiologist, leading to the suggestion by Gleicher and colleagues[15] to form a Gynecoradiology Special Interest Group as a section within the American Fertility Society.

TSS can be performed immediately after an HSG has demonstrated the presence of either unilateral or bilateral proximal tubal obstruction. The transcervical approach to the intramural and isthmic tubal segments is much less invasive than tubocornual anastomosis. TSS is capable of restoring patency to non-occlusive proximal tubal injection failures caused by spasm, debris and filmy adhesions[16]. Capitanio and coworkers[17] used the technique in 108 women who had proximal tubal obstruction (59 unilateral, 49 bilateral) on HSG. Under fluoroscopy, after paracervical block, a repeat HSG is performed. If proximal tubal obstruction is confirmed, a 4.5-F (1.5-mm) catheter is inserted through an 8-F (2.7-mm) introducer and wedged into the tubal ostium, then advanced to the tubal isthmus. If an obstruction is not met, the coaxial guidewire is passed through the catheter. The catheter is advanced over the guidewire, the guidewire is then removed, and 2–3 mL of contrast material injected to verify canalization. The contralateral tube is treated with the same procedure. A conventional HSG is carried out at the end of the TSS procedure. The entire process requires less than 1 min for each tube. In 108 women, 155 tubes were catheterized whereas 9 could not be catheterized. Of the 146 successfully treated tubes, 110 became patent, 21 showed distal occlusion, 10 showed partial distal occlusion and the remaining 5 showed midtubal obstruction; there were two cases of tubal perforation. Of the 46 women who had 'successful' tubal canalization, only 4 achieved term pregnancies and none had tubal pregnancies.

In most series, the obstructed tube can be catheterized and tubal patency demonstrated in more than 80% of patients[18-22]. Thus, tubocornual anastomosis has become a relatively infrequent operation and the standard of care dictates that, in women undergoing HSG or at laparoscopy, TSS is essential prior to tubal microsurgery or IVF. In an attempt to standardize HSG and TSS, Gleicher and colleagues[6] measured tubal perfusion pressures during TSS and correlated them with tubal opacification. The authors noted a wide range of pressures (429 ± 376 mmHg) which was significantly lower than that seen in abnormal-looking tubes (957 ± 445 mmHg). These results suggest that the concomitant performance of perfusion pressure studies during TSS enhanced its capability to detect abnormalities in the Fallopian tubes.

Predictive value

Another variation of non-operative tubal patency studies was reported by Tufekci and coworkers[23], who performed transvaginal sonosalpingography (TVSOS) using 10–20 mL of isotonic saline injected into the uterine cavity through a catheter. In 39 women, TVSOS accurately showed patency in 29 patients and bilateral non-patency in 3. When compared with laparoscopy in 10 women, the results were partially confirmed. Intratubal flow was followed for 5 s through each tube and fimbrial turbulence or cul-de-sac fluid accumulation was considered evidence of patency of at least one tube. TVSOS indicated patency or non-patency of one or both tubes in 37 of 38 patients. The results were confirmed by subsequent chromotubation at laparoscopy with 1% methylene blue. The advantages over HSG claimed by the authors were its greater potential safety, greater convenience and lower cost, its lack of potential interaction with contrast media, and the fact that it is a simple postoperative test following tubal anastomosis.

Both HSG and laparoscopy have some predictability as regards pregnancy outcome following microsurgical neosalpingostomy[24-36]. On HSG, the mucosal pattern as evidenced by the presence or absence of the dark line in the ampulla, and the diameter of the hydrosalpinx and its expansibility are characteristics to be sought in evaluating the salpingogram. The most important feature is the radiological character of the mucosal pattern. During laparoscopy or laparotomy, the extent and nature of the adhesions, the thickness of the tubal wall and the diameter of the hydrosalpinx affect the postoperative prognosis for fertility (Table 13.1).

Opsahl and colleagues[27] performed laparoscopy in 756 patients at 2–9 months after HSG and noted that a normal HSG was confirmed at laparoscopy in 326 of 327 patients, a 96.6% accuracy. In abnormal tubes, 89 of 93 HSGs were confirmed at laparoscopy. The largest differences between the findings of the two tests was in the 336 HSGs with equivocal findings. Moderate-to-severe non-pelvic disease can occur occasionally in women despite a normal HSG and, thus, laparoscopy should be performed in such patients when other factors have been corrected, but pregnancy has not occurred. Salpingograms with equivocal findings should be confirmed by laparoscopy because the radiological results could be false-positive (proximal tubal obstruction caused by spasm or debris) or there may be significant pelvic disease. The distally obstructed tubes in certain instances are not amenable to operative repair and, in other situations, the prognosis for pregnancy postoperatively is so low that patients should be spared even a laparoscopy and entered directly into an IVF or adoption program.

Although many gynecologists use HSG as a screening procedure to establish tubal

Table 13.1 Predictive value of hysterosalpingography and laparoscopy in hydrosalpinx

Hysterosalpingogram
Mucosal pattern
Diameter of hydrosalpinx
Expansibility of ampulla

Laparoscopy
Extent and type of periadnexal adhesions
Thickness of tubal wall
Diameter of hydrosalpinx

disease preoperatively, few studies have been carried out to assess its sensitivity and specificity following tubal microsurgery. Letterie and coworkers[28] correlated HSG and laparoscopy findings after tubal anastomosis in 11 patients and following distal salpingostomies in 14 patients. HSG was able to assess accurately the presence of tubal patency, but was limited in its ability to detect tubal adhesions. Thus, a screening HSG should be performed in the postoperative patient who has not achieved a pregnancy within 6 months. If recurrent tubal occlusion is noted, then IVF is advised but, if patency is seen, then another 6 months should elapse before a repeat laparoscopy is indicated to search for periadnexal adhesions.

HSG should be used preoperatively in planning a myomectomy because the contours of the uterine cavity can be observed and the patency of the Fallopian tubes ascertained[29]. Postoperatively, a search can be made of the cavity for intrauterine adhesions or myometrial defects and the impact of the operation on the Fallopian tubes reassessed. Another possible use of HSG is in the early differential diagnosis of an intrauterine pregnancy from an intratubal abortion in patients who have declining or low levels of human chorionic gonadotropin (hCG). Of four patients in whom transvaginal sonography could not confirm pregnancy, three showed the characteristic finding of a tubal pregnancy on HSG. A normal-looking uterine cavity with the finding of a small saccular diverticulum arising from the tubal isthmus is apparently diagnostic whereas, in contrast, a missed intrauterine abortion shows a characteristic abnormal uterine cavity[30]. In association with low positive hCG titers and an apparently normal uterine cavity, this radiological picture should suggest a strong suspicion that an early tubal pregnancy has occurred. HSG studies should only be performed after the hCG values have declined significantly. It is suggested that HSG be performed in patients who have so-called biochemical pregnancy losses and a history of tubal disease or previous tubal surgery. The clinical implications for the patient who has radiological evidence of a tubal pregnancy is that she is likely to have another tubal pregnancy.

Summary

Hysterosalpingography remains an excellent screening examination to search for intrauterine and tubal causes of infertility (Table 13.2). The findings can avoid the need for laparoscopy in some patients with advanced tubal abnormalities. In selected cases, HSG can be therapeutic, as suggested by the results of the use of oil-soluble media in patients with unexplained infertility and the use of interventional coaxial tubal catheterization for proximal tubal obstruction. Laparoscopy (Table 3.3) is both diagnostic and therapeutic, and has a wide range of applications requiring minimally invasive surgery. The use of these two procedures is to be considered essential in the management of the infertile patient.

Table 13.2 Hysterosalpingography as a screen for intrauterine and tubal causes of infertility

Uterine cavity
Normal triangular shape
Congenital uterine anomalies
Intrauterine adhesions
Submucosal tumors
  polyps / myomas

Fallopian tubes
Diagnostically
  normal fill and spill
  intramural polyps
  salpingitis isthmica nodosa
  endometriosis / tuberculosis
  hydrosalpinx
    operability
    prognosis for fertility
Therapeutically
  normal Fallopian tubes
    use of OBCM for fertility enhancement
  proximal tubal obstruction
    selective salpingography and cannulation

Accuracy
Excellent for uterine cavity disease screening
Screening for Fallopian tube disease
  normal
  suspicious
  abnormal
Poor for endometriosis / periadnexal disease screening

Common errors
Failure to opacify entire uterine cavity
  axial view
  failed cervical traction
  balloon-catheter technique
  opaque vaginal speculum
Failure to evaluate Fallopian tubes properly
  endpoints fill / spill or
  increased abdominal pain / intravasation
  no drainage film
  mucosal pattern obscured

Table 13.3 Features of laparoscopy

Diagnostic value
Detects endometriosis
Locates periadnexal adhesions
Examines uterus
  serosal surface only
Evaluates tubes
  serosal surface, consistency, delineation
    of fimbria

Therapeutic role
Endometriosis
Lyses periadnexal adhesions
Neosalpingostomy
Monitors hysteroscopic cannulation
?Tubal anastomosis for reversal of tubal sterilization
?Myomectomy in selected instances

References

1. Yoder IC, Hall DA. Hysterosalpingography in the 1990s. *Am J Radiol* 1991;157:675–83

2. Hugh AE. The role of hysterosalpingography in modern gynecological practice. *Br J Radiol* 1993;66:278–9

3. Hunt RB, Siegler AM. *Hysterosalpingography: Techniques and Interpretation.* Chicago: Year Book Medical, 1990

4. Angtuaco TL, Boyd CM, London SN, *et al.* Technetium-99 hysterosalpingography in infertility: An accurate alternative to contrast hysterosalpingography. *Radiographics* 1989;9: 115–28

5. Jacobson A, Uszler JM. A simplified technique for radionuclide hysterosalpingography. *J Assist Reprod Genet* 1993;10:4–10

6. Gleicher N, Parrilli M, Redding L, *et al.* Standardization of hysterosalpingography and selective salpingography: A valuable adjunct to simple opacification studies. *Fertil Steril* 1992;58:1136–41

7. Hofman GE, Scott RT, Rosenwaks Z. Common technical errors in hysterosalpingography. *Int J Fertil* 1992;37:41–3

8. Letterie GS, Rose GS. Pregnancy rates after the use of oil-based and water-based contrast media to evaluate tubal patency. *South Med J* 1990;83:1402–3

9. Rasmussen F, Lindequist S, Larsen C, *et al.* Therapeutic effect of hysterosalpingography: Oil- versus water-soluble contrast media, a randomized prospective study. *Radiology* 1991;179:75–8

10. Goodman SB, Rein MS, Hill JA. Hysterosalpingography contrast media and chromopertubation dye inhibit peritoneal lymphocyte and macrophage function in vitro: A potential mechanism for fertility enhancement. *Fertil Steril* 1993;59:1022–7

11. Lisse K, Sydow P. Fallopian tube catheterization and recanalization under ultrasonic observation: A simplified technique to evaluate tubal patency and open proximally obstructed tubes. *Fertil Steril* 1991;56: 198–203

12. Martensson O, Nilsson B, Ekelund L, *et al.* Selective salpingography and fluoroscopic transcervical salpingoplasty for diagnosis and treatment of proximal tube occlusions. *Acta Obstet Gynecol Scand* 1993;72:458–64

13. Isaacson KB, Amendola M, Banner B, *et al.* Transcervical fallopian tube recanalization: a safe and effective therapy for patients with proximal tubal obstruction. *Int J Fertil* 1992; 37:106–10

14. Thurmond AS, Rosch J. Nonsurgical fallopian tube recanalization for treatment of infertility. *Radiology* 1990;174:371–4

15. Gleicher N, Thurmond AS, Burry KA, *et al.* Gynecoradiology: A new approach to diagnosis and treatment of tubal disease. *Fertil Steril* 1992;58:885–7

16. Sulak PJ, Letterie GS, Coddington CC, *et al.* Histology of proximal tubal occlusion. *Fertil Steril* 1987;48:437–40

17. Capitanio GL, Ferraiolo A, Croce S, et al. Transcervical selective salpingography: A diagnostic and therapeutic approach to cases of proximal tubal obstruction. Fertil Steril 1991;55:1045–50

18. Confino E, Tur-Kaspa I, DeCherney A, et al. Transcervical balloon tuboplasty: A multi-center study. J Am Med Assoc 1990;264: 2079–82

19. Burke P, Sabia A, Di Virgilio MR, et al. Indications for tubal recanalisation in diagnostic and interventional hysterosalpingography. Radiol Med 1993;85:657–61

20. Kumpe DA, Zwerdlinger SC, Rothbarth LJ, et al. Proximal fallopian tube occlusion: Diagnosis and treatment with transcervical fallopian tube catheterization. Radiology 1990;177:183–7

21. Lang EK, Dunaway HE Jr, Roniger WE. Selective osteal salpingography and trans-cervical catheter dilatation in the diagnosis and treatment of fallopian tube obstruction. Am J Radiol 1990;154:735–8

22. Lederer KJ. Transcervical tubal cannulation and salpingoscopy in the treatment of tubal infertility. Curr Opin Obstet Gynecol 1993; 5:240–4

23. Tufekci EC, Girit S, Bayirli E, et al. Evaluation of tubal patency by transvaginal sonosalpingography. Fertil Steril 1992;57:336–40

24. Henig I, Prough SG, Cheatwood M, et al. Hysterosalpingography, laparoscopy and hysteroscopy in infertility. A comparative study. J Reprod Med 1991;36:573–5

25. te Velde ER, Boer-Meisel ME, Meisner J, et al. The significance of preoperative hysterosalpingography and laparoscopy for predicting pregnancy outcome in patients with a bilateral hydrosalpinx. Eur J Obstet Gynecol Reprod Biol 1989;31:33–45

26. Schnack Peen UB, Pelle J, Bostofte E, et al. Hysterosalpingography, pre- and postoperative laparoscopy in operative treatment of infertility. Acta Eur Fertil 1989;20:355–8

27. Opsahl MS, Miller B, Klein TA. The predictive value of hysterosalpingography for tubal and peritoneal infertility factors. Fertil Steril 1993; 60:444–8

28. Letterie GS, Haggerty MF, Fellows DW. Sensitivity of hysterosalpingography after tubal surgery. Arch Gynecol Obstet 1992; 251:175–80

29. Karasick S, Ehrlich S. The value of hysterosalpingography before reversal of sterilization procedures involving the fallopian tubes. Am J Radiol 1989;153:1247–50

30. Gleicher N, Parilli M, Pratt DE. Hysterosalpingography and selective salpingography in the differential diagnosis of chemical intrauterine versus tubal pregnancy. Fertil Steril 1993;57:553–8

14 An introduction to gynecological ultrasonography

Leeber Cohen

During the last decade, it has become increasingly common for gynecologists to perform office and emergency-room ultrasound procedures. Although there is controversy surrounding training and credentialing, the need for a basic understanding of the instrumentation and principles of gynecological ultrasonography is clear. This has been best demonstrated by the rapid and accurate evaluation of suspect ectopic pregnancy in the emergency-room setting using transvaginal ultrasound (TVS)[1].

TVS, which is usually performed with an empty bladder, allows the clinician to image the uterus and adnexa to a high degree of resolution at the time of pelvic examination. This is particularly helpful in obese women and patients with abdominal guarding where pelvic examination is difficult. Common causes of menorrhagia, such as polyps and submucous leiomyomata, can be evaluated, and the risk for endometrial hyperplasia or endometrial cancer in women with postmenopausal bleeding determined by measuring the endometrial stripe. Suspect adnexal masses on bimanual examination can be visualized and the appropriate management determined.

Instrumentation

The usual ultrasound machine for the gynecological office comes equipped with a 3.5-mHz curvilinear transabdominal probe and a 7.5-mHz transvaginal probe. Color Doppler (CDI) and cine-loop capabilities add substantially to the cost of the machine, although such options are not necessary unless experts who can perform fetal echocardiography and level-two obstetric ultrasound are available. The need for CDI in gynecological ultrasonography remains controversial and is not an established part of the usual office setting.

The initial setup should be carried out by a qualified applications specialist sent by the manufacturer. The software to run the machine should be installed such that the SPTA (spatial peak temporal average) power limit of $100\,mW/cm^2$ cannot be exceeded. Presettings for preprocessing, postprocessing, focus zones and filters should be set so that a minimum of adjustment is required by the practitioner. If these concepts are unfamiliar, the practitioner is encouraged to attend a course or read one of the basic texts[2].

Major advantages and disadvantages of the transabdominal and transvaginal probes compared with each other should be emphasized. The 3.5-mHz curvilinear probe is designed to give a wide-angle view (150°) of the pelvis; its lower frequency allows visualization of structures located up to 14 cm from the transducer. Masses that are large or located high in the pelvis should be evaluated by transabdominal ultrasound. The 7.5-mHz transvaginal probe yields a 90° view and can visualize structures close to the vaginal apex with a high degree of resolution. However, there is rapid attenuation of sound, and structures lying > 8 cm away are poorly seen. Not all cases require the use of both types of ultrasound although, occasionally, both techniques may be necessary. Good clinical judgment and experience are certainly required.

The first session that a resident spends in the department should be devoted to familiarization with the equipment, and a review of the involved physics and procedures. The session should include the proper attachment and removal of transducers to avoid damage to the connecting pins. Proper cleansing of transducers and sterilization of vaginal probes must be emphasized. Glutaraldehyde (Cidex™) can be used for a minimum of 15 min to clean the vaginal probes between examinations. Probe covers or condoms are required for the vaginal probe. A gel or lubricant interface is to be used both inside and outside the probe cover for proper transmission of sound.

The physician should be familiar with the location of the on-off switch, overall-gain control, fine-gain controls [time-gain compensation (TGC) toggles] and magnification controls, and the measurement software. The patient's name should be placed at the beginning of the examination and all pictures well labeled. As orientation varies from one institution to another, pictures should be labeled 'longitudinal', 'transverse', 'left' and 'right'.

Orientation

The most difficult concept to teach in gynecological ultrasound is orientation. Both the ultrasound probe and image must be orientated so as to allow the practitioner to interpret the image correctly. Most ultrasound laboratories in the USA orientate the front of the transducer to the left side of the screen (Figure 14.1). Most machines designate this orientation by an arrow or symbol at the top of the screen. For transabdominal ultrasound, most ultrasound units in the USA image longitudinal midline pictures with the patient's bladder showing on the right side of the screen, accomplished by aiming the front of the transducer, indicated on the transducer by a longitudinal groove or label, towards

the patient's head. If the bladder does not appear on the right side of the screen (see Figure 14.1), the left–right inverse switch needs to be changed. For transverse images (Figure 14.2), the front of the transducer is aimed to the patient's right; the patient's left

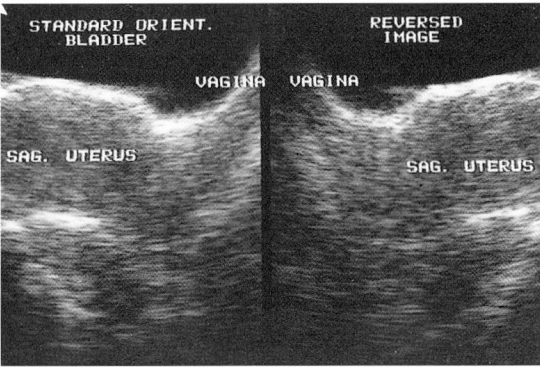

Figure 14.1 Transabdominal longitudinal images. Standard orientation used in the USA (left): The front of the transducer is imaged on the left and the inferior aspect of the bladder is on the right. In the non-standard orientation (right), the image is rotated 180° by orientating the front of the transducer to the right side of the image

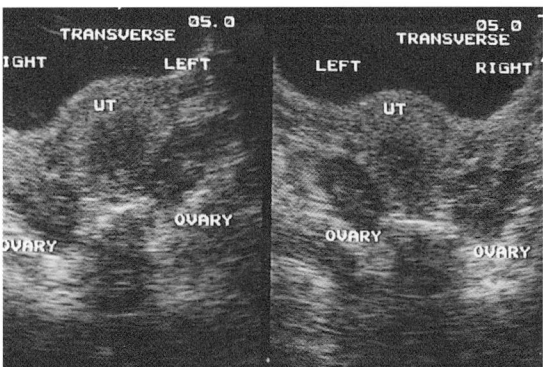

Figure 14.2 Transabdominal transverse images. In the standard orientation used by most radiologists in the USA (left), the front of the transducer is imaged on the left side of the screen; the patient's right side is displayed on the left and the patient's left is on the right. In the non-standard orientation (right), the image can be rotated 180° by reversing the orientation of the transducer (indicated by a little arrow at top of screen)

side will then appear on the right and *vice versa* . The orientation of the probe and the image must be checked at the beginning of each scan and vigilance maintained to avoid accidentally changing it.

Multiple orientations have been suggested for TVS displays. However, most ultrasound centers scan with the front of the vaginal transducer displayed on the left side of the screen. Aiming the front of the transducer at the bladder will result in an image of the bladder on the left side of the screen whereas the cervix or vagina are usually displayed at the top of the image and the uterine fundus inferiorly. Anteversion or retroversion can be determined by the relative position of the uterus to the bladder (Figure 14.3). As the vaginal probe transducer fires from the front end, for transverse images, the transducer needs to be flipped to scan the opposite side. This makes labeling of the images for right and left sides doubly important.

The physician performing a transvaginal scan needs to be aware of the increased

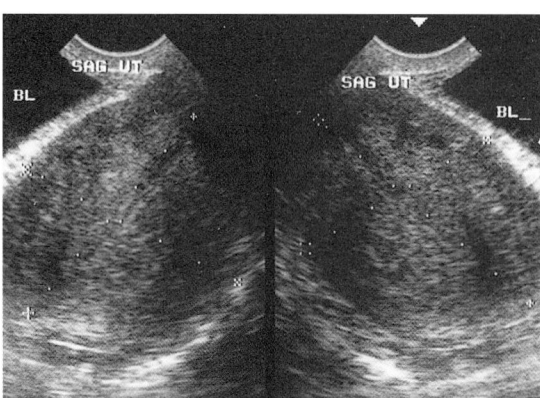

Figure 14.3 Many ultrasound laboratories orientate the front of the transducer to the left side of the screen so that the cervix and vagina are at the top of the image with the uterine fundus below. (Left) The uterus is antroverted (rotated towards the bladder); (right) the same image with the front of the transducer to the right rotates the image 180° along the x axis

anxiety produced by this scan in some women. The length of the probe is potentially alarming, so the depth of insertion and manipulation of the probe should be explained to the patient prior to the examination. With patients who appear to be nervous or have difficulty in relaxing for the examination, it may be better to have them insert the vaginal probe themselves.

If possible, both a physician and a sonographer should be present during the examination, one to perform the transvaginal procedure, the other to adjust and record the images on the machine. One person alone may perform both functions, but this requires practice to avoid any awkwardness. Furthermore, the second person may also serve as a chaperon.

As already mentioned, the vaginal probe should be carefully cleaned prior to use. A probe cover is mandatory. Ultrasound jelly should be applied to the inside of the probe cover and adequate lubricant spread on the outer surfaces. The transducer should be gently introduced in a longitudinal direction. If the bladder has not been completely emptied, the patient should be asked to try again. Images of the cervix, lower uterine segment and fundus should be obtained in both longitudinal and transverse planes, and the adnexa identified. These are usually located between the uterus and the iliac vessels, which serve as a landmark. The adnexa and any masses should be measured in three dimensions. The cul-de-sac should be imaged and the presence of fluid or clot-like echoes noted and measured.

The depth of insertion, plane of the long axis and lateral position of the transducer all require adjustment to achieve proper images of these structures. This is most easily accomplished when the patient's feet are placed in stirrups, thereby allowing adequate abduction of the legs. If stirrups are not available, imaging an anteverted uterus may be difficult, although elevating the patient's hips with a pad or pillow should help.

TVS in clinical situations

Early pregnancy loss and ectopic pregnancy

The evaluation of early pregnancy bleeding and suspected ectopic pregnancy has been greatly eased by the transvaginal probe. The orderly appearance of the gestational sac at 28–35 days, the yolk sac at 35–48 days and the fetal pole at 42–56 days has been demonstrated by Warren and colleagues[3] (Figures 14.4 and 14.5), using transvaginal ultrasound and β-human chorionic gonadotropin (hCG) titers as standardized by the First International Reference Preparation. Discriminatory zones for β-hCG may be 1500 for the gestational sac, 7000 for the yolk sac and 17 000 for the fetal pole with heart beat[4]. As a number of different β-hCG assay kits using three different standard preparations are currently available, practitioners need to establish β-hCG discriminatory zones for each laboratory involved. Ideally, each ultrasound center should have a chemistry laboratory where the β-hCG measurements are performed. Serial titers should not be performed at two different laboratories as the results may then be discrepant.

Two additional important precautions should be taken when interpreting β-hCG titers. Multiple gestation can result in elevated titers that do not correlate with the expected embryonic structures. Patients with complete or incomplete abortion may have titers elevated to above the discriminatory zone for visualizing a gestational sac. Unnecessary operative interventions may occur if the clinician does not consider all of the clinical presentation data, including patient history, and pelvic examination, laboratory and ultrasound findings.

A yolk sac or a 2–3 mm fetal pole is usually seen when the mean intrauterine gestational sac diameter is 10 mm. If the gestational sac has achieved this size and a yolk sac or fetal pole are not seen, then repeat TVS should be repeated within 1 week. If these structures are still not seen, a diagnosis of a missed abortion can be made. A diagnosis of early pregnancy loss can also be made when the mean gestational sac diameter is greater than 20 mm and a fetal pole with

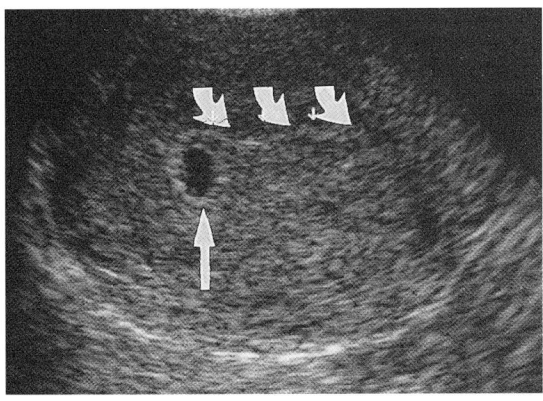

Figure 14.4 Transvaginal picture of a 5-mm early intrauterine gestational sac (straight arrow) is identified adjacent to the endometrial cavity (curved arrows)

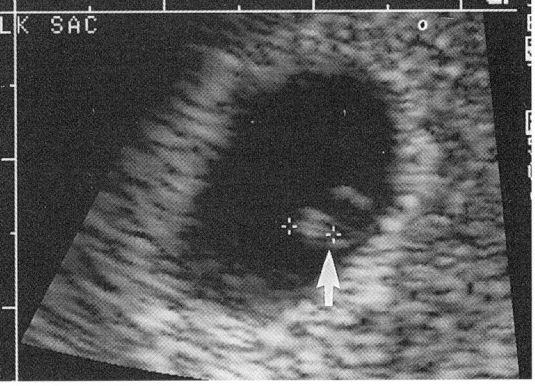

Figure 14.5 Transvaginal image showing a 5-mm yolk sac with an adjacent 3-mm fetal pole (straight arrow)

cardiac activity is not seen[5]. The diagnosis of a missed abortion can also be made by TVS when a fetal pole ≥5 mm fails to exhibit cardiac activity[6].

In women with first trimester bleeding, subchorionic bleeds are frequently identified on ultrasonography. Although the published literature is scanty, it is generally accepted that the larger the bleed, the greater the likelihood of eventual miscarriage (Figure 14.6).

Timor-Tritsch and colleagues[1] have noted that ectopic pregnancies can be properly diagnosed with TVS in the emergency-room setting with a high degree of certainty. In approximately 30% of cases, the ectopic gestational sac can be visualized (Figure 14.7). In the remainder, the absence of an intrauterine gestational sac and the presence of a complex adnexal mass or hemoperitoneum allow the diagnosis of ectopic pregnancy with a high degree of accuracy. Care must be taken not to confuse a cystic corpus luteum with an ectopic gestational sac (Figure 14.8).

It may be difficult to differentiate an early intrauterine gestational sac from a pseudogestational sac, which can be seen in some ectopic pregnancies. The pseudoges-tational sac represents an accumulation of fluid or blood within the decidualized endometrium (Figure 14.9). In patients with minimal peritoneal findings, serial quantitative β-hCG titers and repeat transvaginal scans at 48–72-h intervals are required to make the diagnosis.

The diagnosis of complete abortion can be made by ultrasound when the uterine cavity is empty and one of the following criteria is fulfilled:

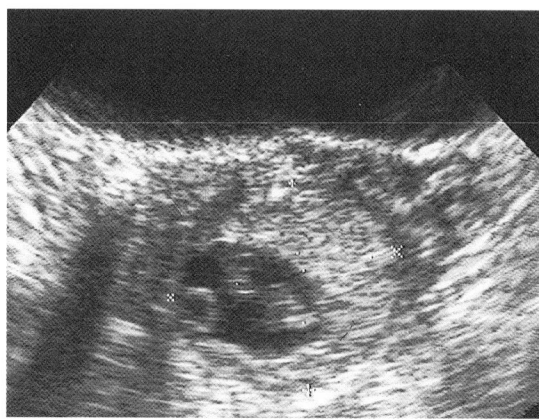

Figure 14.7 Transvaginal image of a tubal pregnancy (3.4×3.0 cm) with fetal pole and yolk sac

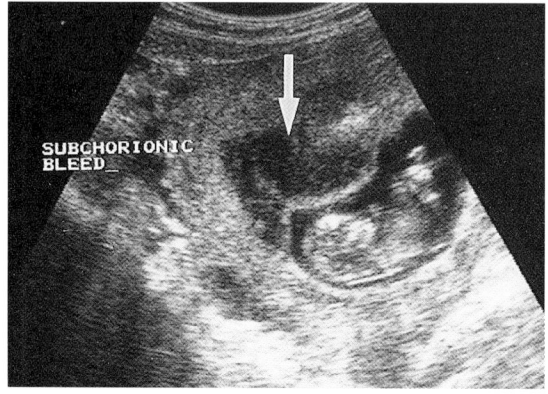

Figure 14.6 Transvaginal image showing a subchorionic bleed, identified by hypoechoic echoes, dissecting between the chorion and uterine wall (straight arrow)

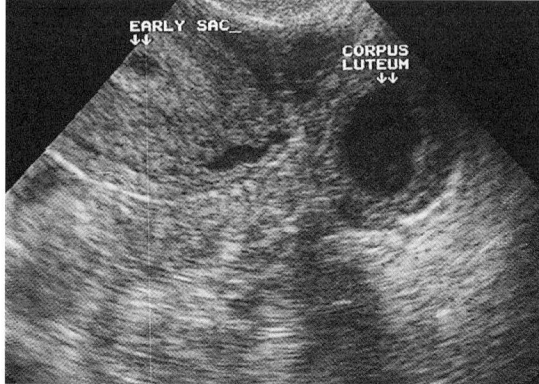

Figure 14.8 Transvaginal image displaying a cystic corpus luteum and early intrauterine gestational sac. The corpus luteum is easily confused with an ectopic gestation

(1) The uterine cavity appears empty and serial β-hCG quantitative titers are rapidly falling towards negative. Initially, the titers should be taken at 48-h intervals;

(2) An intrauterine pregnancy had been demonstrated on an earlier ultrasound, but the uterine cavity is now empty;

(3) Pathology reveals the presence of products of conception.

Failure to meet any of these criteria can lead to the diagnosis of ectopic pregnancy being missed. The rare phenomenon of heterotopic pregnancy, which is becoming more common with assisted reproduction, should not be forgotten.

Functional and hemorrhagic ovarian cysts

Most functional cysts appear to be predominantly cystic and are usually <6 cm in diameter. The cysts usually disappear spontaneously after 1–2 menstrual cycles with or without the use of contraception pills[7].

Hemorrhagic cysts vary widely in echo patterns. These cysts may contain low-level

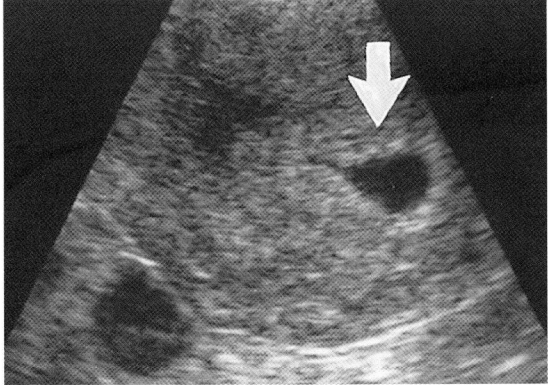

Figure 14.9 Transvaginal image of a pseudogestational sac, which represents a collection of fluid within the decidualized endometrial cavity

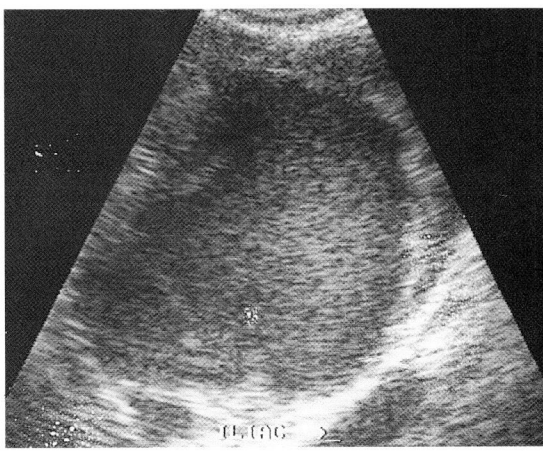

Figure 14.10 Transvaginal image of an endometrioma. Approximately 60–70% of endometriotic cysts are filled with low-level echoes, a pattern which is also seen in hemorrhagic cysts and abscesses

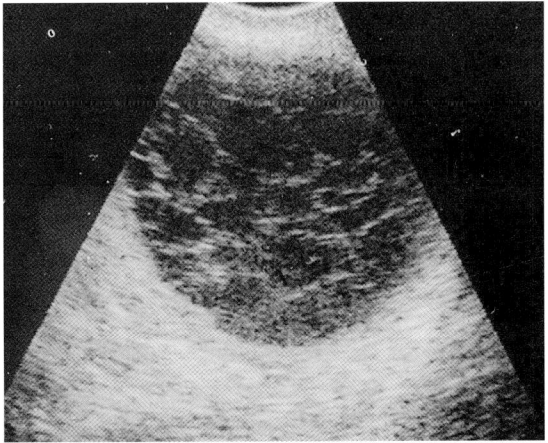

Figure 14.11 Transvaginal image of a resolving hemorrhagic corpus luteum shows a cribriform pattern of low-level echoes within the cyst. These masses usually spontaneously resolve within 4–8 weeks

internal echoes, thereby mimicking the pattern typically associated with endometriosis (Figures 14.10–14.13), or areas of scattered low-level internal echogenicity, which are also seen in endometriomas or mucinous neoplasms[8], or areas of dense echogenicity, thereby resembling cystic tera-

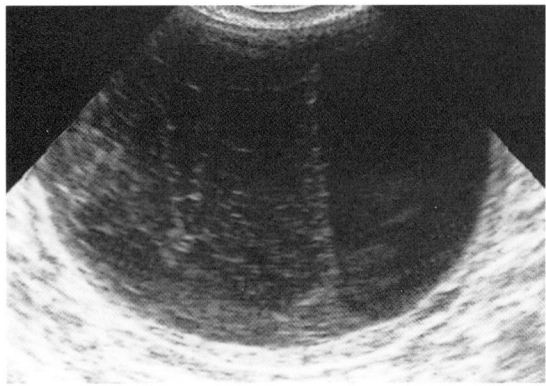

Figure 14.12 Transvaginal image of a resolving hemorrhagic corpus luteum showing low-level internal echoes within the cyst. An old endometrioma may present an identical appearance

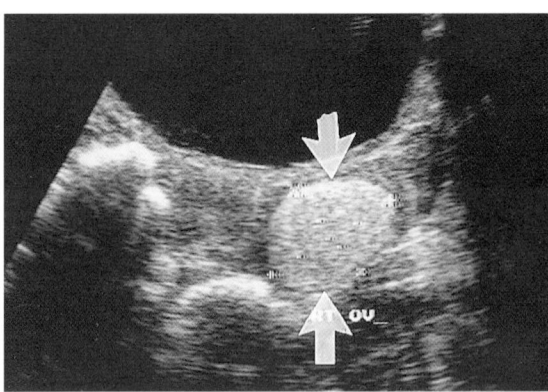

Figure 14.14 Transabdominal image showing a densely echogenic cystic teratoma

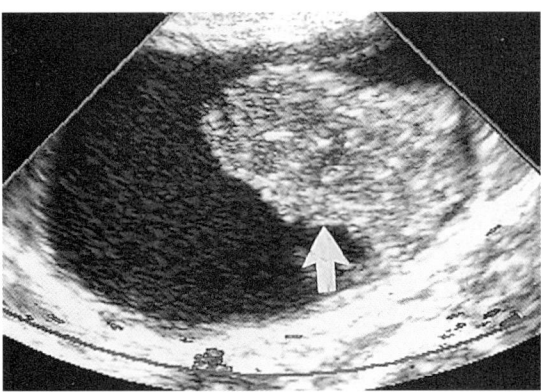

Figure 14.13 Transvaginal image of a complex mass with a papillary-like internal projection. Pathology revealed a corpus luteum; the echogenic material (arrow) was clotted blood. A cystic teratoma or papillary adenocarcinoma may present an identical image

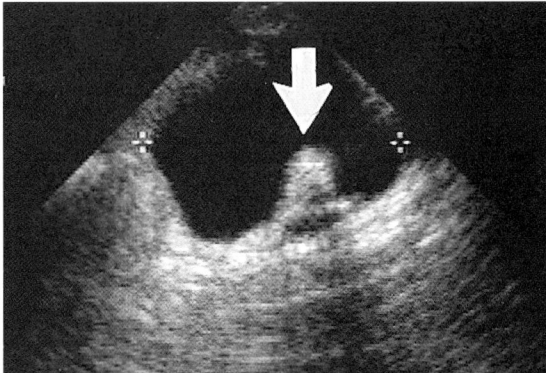

Figure 14.15 Transvaginal image of a cystic teratoma with a large cystic component and a papillary-like projection with posterior shadowing (arrow). The echo pattern of cystic teratomas is frequently complex and can render differentiation from malignant tumors difficult

tomas or malignant neoplasms. Fortunately, most hemorrhagic cysts spontaneously disappear within 1–2 menstrual cycles.

Ovarian neoplasms

Ultrasound attributes associated with a high probability of benign disease include a mass that is < 8 cm or cystic, minimally septated or with no solid areas[9]. However, in premenopausal women, dermoid cysts are the excep-

tion to these characteristics. Some workers believe that these masses can be preoperatively identified by their characteristic dense echogenicity and posterior shadowing (Figures 14.14 and 14.15)[10,11]. A higher index for suspected ovarian malignancy should be considered if a neoplasm is found in a postmenopausal woman; a mass > 8 cm, multiseptations and solid areas within a neoplasm are all associated with a higher risk of malignancy (Figures 14.16 and 14.17). Many

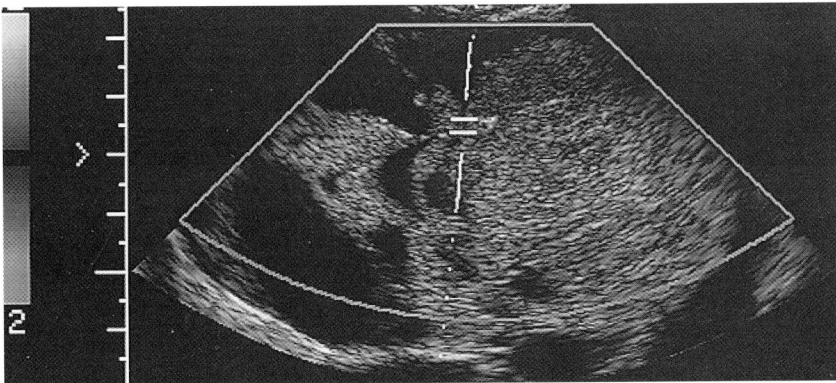

Figure 14.16 Transvaginal image of a complex papillary serous adeno-carcinoma with cystic spaces alternating with solid elements. Color Doppler revealed neovascularization within the tumor

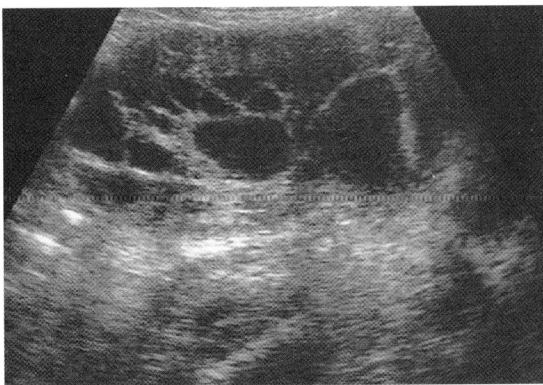

Figure 14.17 Image of a multiseptated mucinous adenocarcinoma

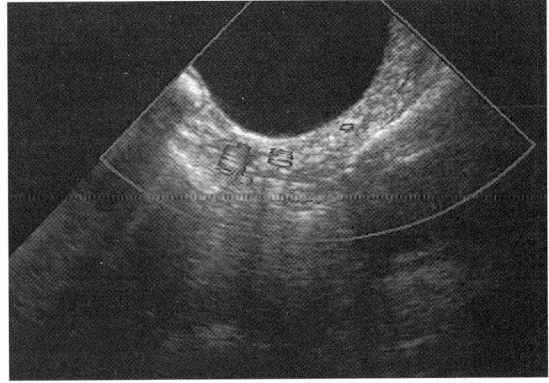

Figure 14.18 Transvaginal image of a thin-walled 4.5-cm cyst in a postmenopausal woman shows no septations, solid areas or neovascularization

laboratories use the transvaginal scoring system of Sassone and colleagues[12] to assess the risk of malignancy in an adnexal mass.

The inexperienced sonologist is advised to seek second opinions when an adnexal mass is found during an ultrasound examination although, even with years of ultrasound experience, it is an imperfect art. There is much overlap in premenopausal women of the appearances of functional cysts, endometriomas and hemorrhagic cysts on ultrasound. A combination of repeat history, pelvic examination and ultrasound is often required to correctly identify the presence or absence of pathology.

Similarly, in postmenopausal women, the presence of a cystic mass <6 cm does not necessarily indicate that the patient requires surgery (Figure 14.18). Such a finding is seen in 2–3% of postmenopausal women[13] and, in many centers, these women have been followed by repeat examination and measurement of CA-125 tumor marker levels at 6-month intervals; surgery is only performed if clinically indicated.

Dysfunctional bleeding

Transvaginal ultrasonography allows rapid evaluation of uterine size, contour and cavity. The presence of myomas is usually easily established as the echo density and capsules of these tumors usually differ markedly from that of normal uterine tissue[14]. Particular attention should be paid to centrally located leiomyomas which may be submucous or to leiomyomas that appear to impinge on the cavity of the uterus as these tumors are a major cause of abnormal uterine bleeding (Figures 14.19 and 14.20). The clinician should also remember that adenomyosis can cause heavy irregular periods, but is frequently not obvious on transvaginal scanning. The best clues are diffuse uterine enlargement, absence of myoma-like echoes and, occasionally, visualization of glandular spaces in the uterine wall.

The endometrial cavity is easily identified and submucous leiomyomas readily mapped when a secretory endometrium is present. When the clinician has become more experienced with the ultrasound technique, sonohysterography in the office setting may provide improved visualization of the uterine cavity. For the hysteroscopic surgeon to be successful, the depth of penetration of the submucous leiomyoma in the uterine wall must be appreciated.

Postmenopausal bleeding

Although endometrial biopsy remains the gold standard for evaluation of postmenopausal bleeding, TVS can be used to assess the risk for endometrial malignancy in these patients. Karlsson and colleagues[15] studied a large series of 1168 women with postmenopausal bleeding, 114 of whom had endometrial cancer, and demonstrated that the endometrial stripe should be ≤4 mm in postmenopausal women not receiving hormone replacement therapy (HRT; Figure 14.21). In a study by Zalud and coworkers[16] in postmenopausal women taking continuous HRT

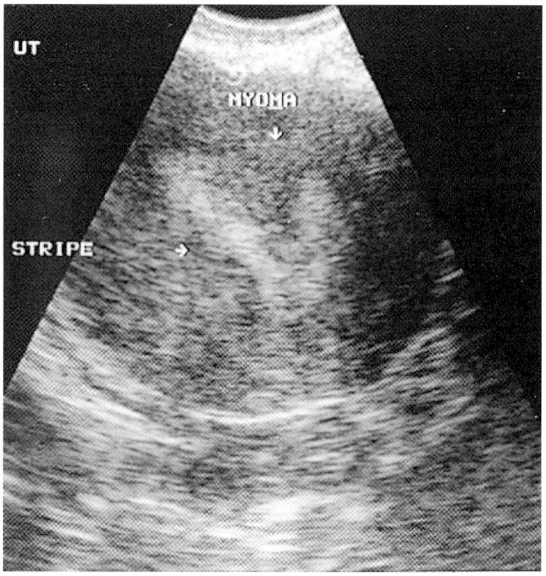

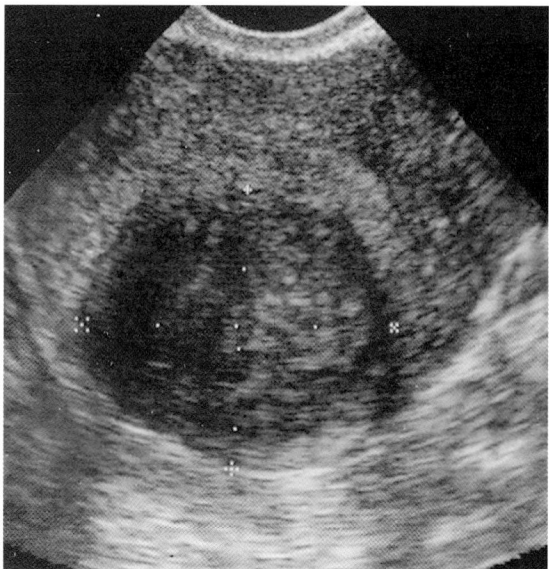

Figure 14.19 Transvaginal image of a submucous leiomyoma that is clearly seen surrounded by a secretory endometrium

Figure 14.20 Transvaginal image of an intramural leiomyoma extending from the endometrial mucosa to the uterine serosa

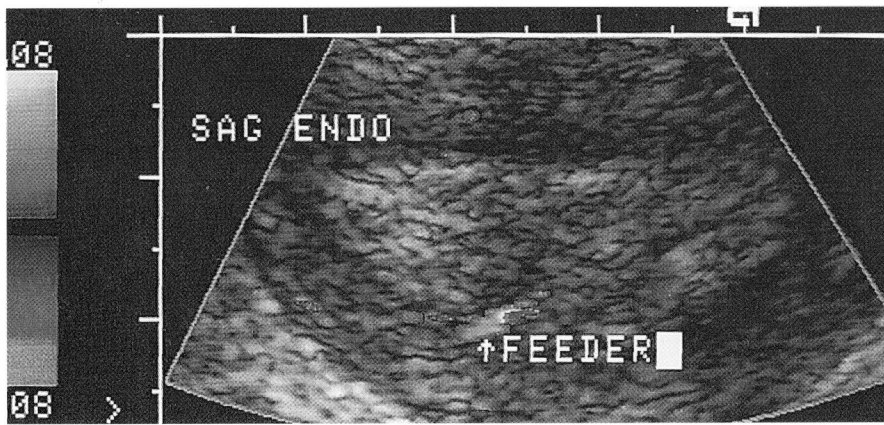

Figure 14.21 Transvaginal image from a postmenopausal woman with an endometrium thickened to 12 mm. Color Doppler revealed a vascular structure entering the uterine cavity. The patient had a minimally invasive adenocarcinoma

[conjugated estrogen (Premarin® 0.625 mg) and medroxyprogesterone acetate (Provera® 2.5 mg) daily], the investigators found that the average ±1 standard deviation endometrial thickness was 7.6 + 2.6 mm. Bonilla-Musoles and colleagues[17], using a different form of continuous HRT regimen [Estraderm TTS® (patch) and Provera 2.5 mg], found an average endometrial thickness of 4.2 (range 0–14) mm. These investigators also reported an average endometrial thickness of 6.6 (range 2–15) mm with sequential therapy (Estraderm TTS and Provera 10 mg on days 17–28 of the cycle)[17]. Lin and coworkers[18] demonstrated an average endometrial stripe of 6 ±3.9 (range 0.1–17) mm in women taking cyclical therapy (Premarin 0.625–1.25 mg on cycle days 1–25 and Provera 5 or 10 mg on the last 10–13 days of estrogen therapy). It has not been established in the literature whether it is safe to use a >5-mm endometrial thickness cut-off point in women with irregular postmenopausal bleeding receiving HRT.

Tamoxifen effects

Tamoxifen can lead to thickening of the endometrium in both pre- and postmenopausal women. Large endometrial polyps may be seen with use of this medication (Figure 14.22). The endometrial stripe may be difficult to measure in postmenopausal women due to the appearance of subepithelial lucencies. In the presence of irregular bleeding, a sonohysterogram or hysteroscopy in addition to biopsy may be required to evaluate these patients. Tamoxifen can also lead to hyperstimulation of the ovary, particularly in premenopausal patients (Figure 14.23).

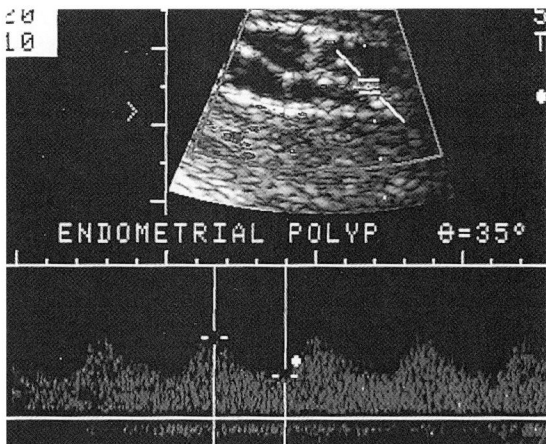

Figure 14.22 Transvaginal image of a complex vascular polyp in a postmenopausal woman receiving tamoxifen treatment for breast cancer

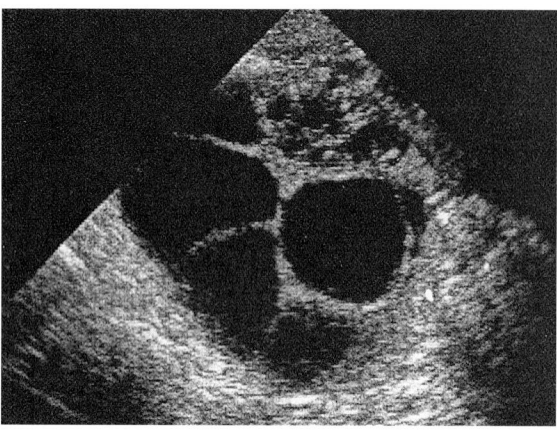

Figure 14.23 Transvaginal image of a multicystic ovary in a premenopausal woman receiving tamoxifen therapy

References

1. Timor-Tritsch IE, Yeh MN, Peisner DB, *et al.* The use of transvaginal sonography in the diagnosis of ectopic pregnancy. *Am J Obstet Gynecol* 1989;161:157–61

2. Kremkau F. *Diagnostic Ultrasound: Principles, Instruments, and Exercises*, 3rd edn. Philadelphia: WB Saunders, 1989

3. Warren WB, Timor-Tritsch IE, Peisner DB, *et al.* Dating the early pregnancy by sequential appearance of embryonic structures. *Am J Obstet Gynecol* 1989;161:747–53

4. American College of Obstetrics and Gynecology. Ectopic pregnancy. *ACOG Tech Bull* 1990; December (150)

5. Rempen A. Diagnosis of viability in early pregnancy with vaginal sonography. *J Ultrasound Med* 1990;9:711–6

6. Pennell RG, Needleman L, Pajak T, *et al.* Prospective comparison of vaginal and abdominal sonography in normal early pregnancy. *J Ultrasound Med* 1991;10:63–7

7. Steinkampf MP, Hammond KR, Blackwell RE. Hormonal treatment of functional ovarian cysts: A randomized prospective study. *Fertil Steril* 1990;54:775

8. Cohen L, Valle RF, Sabbagha RE. A comparison of the preoperative ultrasound images of surgically proven endometriomas scanned by both transabdominal and transvaginal techniques. *J Gynecol Surg* 1995;11:27–32

9. Maiman M, Seltzer V, Boyce J. Laparoscopic excision of ovarian masses subsequently found to be malignant. *Obstet Gynecol* 1991;77:563–6

10. Mais V, Guerriero S, Ajossa S, *et al.* Transvaginal ultrasonography in the diagnosis of cystic teratoma. *Obstet Gynecol* 1995; 85:48–52

11. Cohen L, Sabbagha R. Echo patterns of benign cystic teratomas by transvaginal ultrasound. *Ultrasound Obstet Gynecol* 1993;3:120–3

12. Sassone AM, Timor-Tritsch IE, Artner A, et al. Transvaginal sonographic characterization of ovarian disease: Evaluation of a new scoring system to predict ovarian malignancy. Obstet Gynecol 1991;78:70–5

13. Goldstein SR, Subramanyam B, Snyder JR, et al. The postmenopausal cystic mass: The potential role of ultrasound in conservative management. Obstet Gynecol 1989;73:8–10

14. Fedele L, Bianchi S, Dorta M, et al. Transvaginal sonography versus hysteroscopy in the diagnosis of uterine submucous myomas. Obstet Gynecol 1991;77:745

15. Karlsson B, Granberg S, Wikland M, et al. Transvaginal ultrasonography of the endometrium in women with postmenopausal bleeding. A Nordic multicenter study. Am J Obstet Gynecol 1995;172:1488–94

16 Zalud I, Conway C, Schulmann H, Trinca D. Endometrial and myometrial thickness and uterine blood flow in postmenopausal women: The influence of hormone replacement and age. J Ultrasound Med 1993;12:737–41

17. Bonilla-Musoles F, Ballester MJ, Marti M, et al. Transvaginal colour Doppler assessment of endometrial status in normal postmenopausal women: The effect of hormone replacement therapy. J Ultrasound Med 1995;14:503–7

18. Lin M, Gosink B, Wolf S, et al. Endometrial thickness after menopause: Effect of hormone replacement. Radiology 1991;180:427–32

15 Computed tomography and magnetic resonance imaging in gynecology

Frederick L. Hoff

Imaging in the evaluation of the female pelvis is dominated by ultrasonography, particularly since the advent of endovaginal techniques. Ultrasound has five principal advantages over other modalities: real-time capability; a multiplane approach; lack of ionizing radiation; relative low cost; and the ability to differentiate between fluid and solid. These advantages allow ultrasound to be the only imaging modality required in many clinical situations. Nevertheless, there are settings in which computed tomography (CT) or magnetic resonance imaging (MRI) can provide additional or unique information which is helpful to the gynecologist.

CTs and MRIs ordered by non-gynecologists in the evaluation of vague or confusing symptoms may indicate a gynecological origin of the symptoms. Also, studies performed to assess unrelated disease may identify incidental pelvic pathology. For these reasons, the gynecologist should not only know when these modalities may be helpful, but should also have a working knowledge of the basics of the procedures and the significance of certain findings. This chapter covers the more frequently encountered abnormalities as well as those situations in which CT and MRI can provide valuable information to the clinician.

Computed tomography

Technique

Conventional CT uses an X-ray tube and a bank of detectors on a rotating gantry to create a digitized cross-sectional image through the patient. This has three implications for the gynecologist: the patient is exposed to ionizing radiation; structures are differentiated only by density; and the images are in an axial orientation. Spiral CT is a relatively new technique which has revolutionized many of the applications of CT. In spiral CT, the X-ray tube and detectors rotate continuously around the patient as she moves through the machine. This allows a much more rapid acquisition of data, all within a single breath-hold. This avoids respiratory variation in slice position and allows for more advantageous use of intravenous contrast material.

Contrast agents are used in CT to alter the density of adjacent structures. Oral contrast is nearly always indicated primarily to prevent a bowel loop from mimicking a cystic adnexal abnormality or adenopathy. Similarly, rectal contrast can distend the rectum and colon to better differentiate pelvic involvement of tumor and infections. Intravenous contrast is also helpful in identifying vascular structures and distinguishing solid masses from fluid.

Normal pelvic CT anatomy

The uterus is routinely visualized as a well-defined muscle-density structure (Figure 15.1 A); however, the amount of useful information is dependent on the uterine position. The endometrium is slightly lower in density than the adjacent myometrium. The cervix is similar in density to the uterus (Figure 15.1 B)

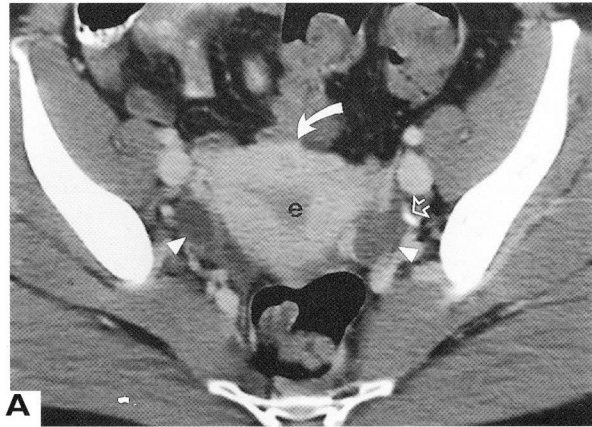

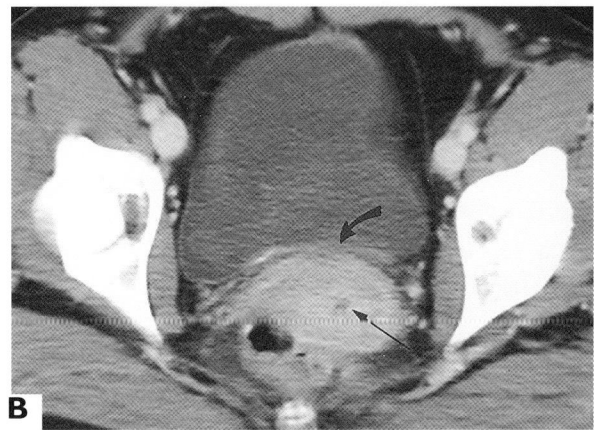

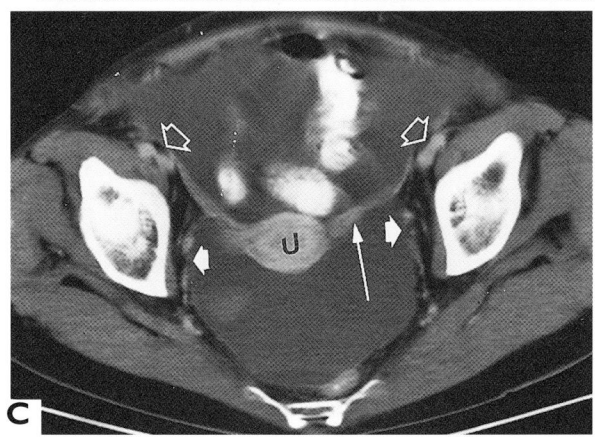

Figure 15.1 Normal CT of the pelvis. (**A**) Axial CT through the pelvis after administration of intravenous contrast demonstrates an anteverted uterus. The fundus (curved arrow) is located anteriorly and a central area of low density represents the endometrium (e). The ovaries are seen laterally (arrowheads). The left ureter is well visualized, being filled with dense contrast (open arrow). (**B**) An image taken more caudally (same patient as in A) demonstrates the cervix (curved arrow) and endocervical canal (arrow); the bladder (arrow) and round ligaments (arrowheads) are located anteriorly. (**C**) The uterus (U) and broad ligaments (long arrow) are well demonstrated by ascites which fills the pelvis. The external (open arrows) and internal (short arrows) iliac vessels are also seen

and is difficult to differentiate from the vaginal fornices surrounding it. The vagina is seen as a collapsed H-shaped structure, and the ovaries appear as heterogeneous structures of soft tissue and fluid density lying just lateral to the uterus (see Figure 15.1 A). The normal Fallopian tubes and broad ligaments are not visualized unless surrounded by ascites (Figure 15.1 C). The round ligaments may occasionally be identified (see Figure 15.1 B).

The surrounding structures of the pelvis are well demonstrated by CT. The common, external and internal iliac arteries and veins are seen in nearly all patients (see Figure 15.1 C). They are easily located in characteristic locations adjacent to the psoas, iliopsoas and obturator internus muscles. The ureter crosses anterior to the iliac artery bifurcation and then courses medially at the level of the sciatic foramen; it can be demonstrated if filled with contrast material (see Figure 15.1 A). Normal lymph nodes are infrequently visualized; they appear as soft tissue-density structures adjacent to the pelvic vessels.

Indications for pelvic CT

There are relatively few specific indications for CT of the female genital tract. Many clinical situations are better evaluated by other means, such as ultrasound and laparoscopy. However, CT can be used to evaluate inflammatory diseases, identify pelvic masses and stage malignancies. Patients who present with acute pain and fever may have inflammatory conditions such as appendicitis, diverticulitis, inflammatory bowel disease or pelvic inflammatory disease. Because clinically these conditions may overlap, CT can be useful in their evaluation, particularly when the results with ultrasound are normal or equivocal. Postoperative patients with possible abscesses are also good candidates for CT; in such patients, ultrasound may often be limited by pain and associated ileus.

Findings on pelvic CT

Uterine fibroid

Uterine leiomyomas are typically hypodense or isodense with the surrounding myometrium (Figure 15.2). Although they are occasionally well-defined, the most common finding is uterine enlargement and a deformed contour[1]. On occasions, it may be difficult to differentiate between a centrally located leiomyoma and endometrial enlargement. The presence of calcification can make identification easier, although only a minority of such lesions contain calcium.

Adnexal findings

Mature teratoma (dermoid cyst)

Most mature teratomas are well-defined masses (Figure 15.3) which often contain multiple elements, including lipid and calcification. A specific diagnosis can be made in up to 98% of cases[2].

Ovarian tumor

Ovarian epithelial tumors generally have both low-density fluid and high-density soft-tissue components (Figures 15.4 and 15.5). These findings in an adnexal mass on CT are non-specific; malignant masses are not reliably differentiated from benign masses, although the presence of wall thickening, septations, papillary projections and solid

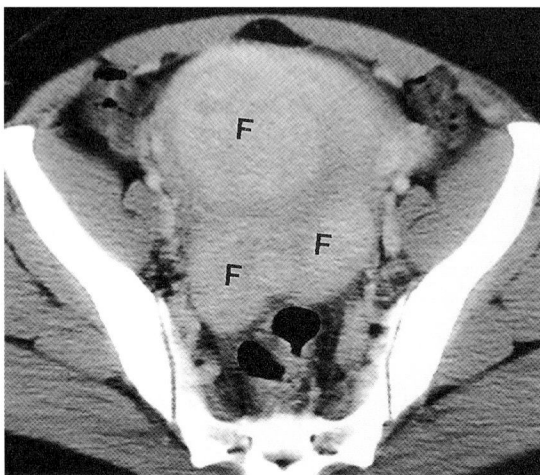

Figure 15.2 Fibroid: Spiral CT through the pelvis obtained during bolus administration of intravenous contrast shows three enhanced uterine fibroids (F)

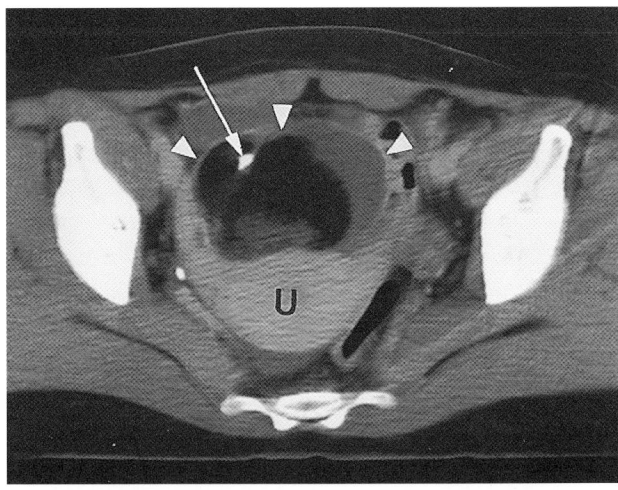

Figure 15.3 Dermoid: CT showing a pelvic mass (arrowheads) to be predominantly fat in density and containing a small area of calcium (arrow), identifying it as a dermoid lying anterior to the uterus (U)

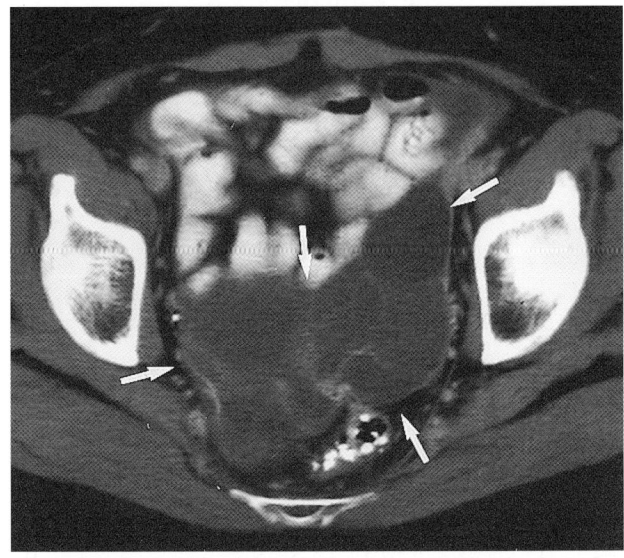

Figure 15.4 Serous cystadenoma: CT showing a lobulated mass (arrows) filling the pelvis to be predominantly fluid in density, and containing multiple thick and thin septa. Although non-specific, the presence of soft-tissue components suggests malignancy. This proved to be a serous cystadenoma on resection

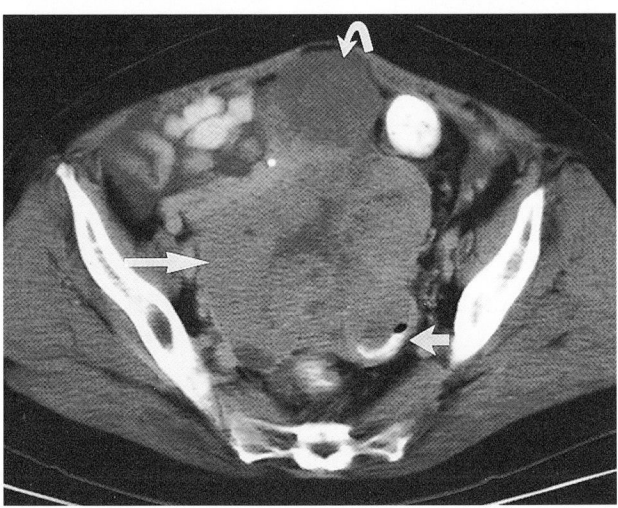

Figure 15.5 Mucinous cystadenocarcinoma: CT showing a large pelvic mass with both solid (arrow) and cystic (curved arrow) components which has invaded the sigmoid colon (short arrow), identified by contrast material and a small amount of air within it

components all suggest malignancy[3]. More important is the capability to preoperatively identify invasion, hydronephrosis, ascites, peritoneal implants and pleural effusions.

Tuboovarian abscess

Abscesses on CT are identified as low-density fluid collections that are often enhanced by a thick-walled rim (Figure 15.6) and an increased density in the adjacent fat. Although non-specific, these findings are highly suggestive in the appropriate clinical setting. CT is particularly useful for atypical cases or when ultrasound is equivocal[4].

Hydro / pyosalpinx

Hydrosalpinx should be suspected whenever a tubular mass is seen in the adnexa on CT (Figure 15.7), in this case, a hematosalpinx.

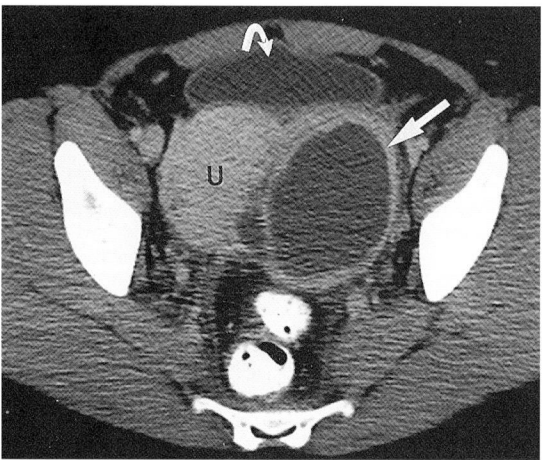

Figure 15.6 Tuboovarian abscess: CT shows that the left adnexa contains a large thick-walled collection of fluid (arrow); the patient had clinical symptoms of pelvic inflammatory disease not responding to antibiotics. This proved to be a tuboovarian abscess. Also labeled are the bladder (curved arrow) and uterus (U), which is displaced to the left by the abscess

The presence of adjacent abnormalities may help to determine the cause and severity.

Miscellaneous findings

Appendicitis

CT is an excellent test in the diagnosis of appendicitis and is preferable, in some centers, to ultrasound. Although its lack of

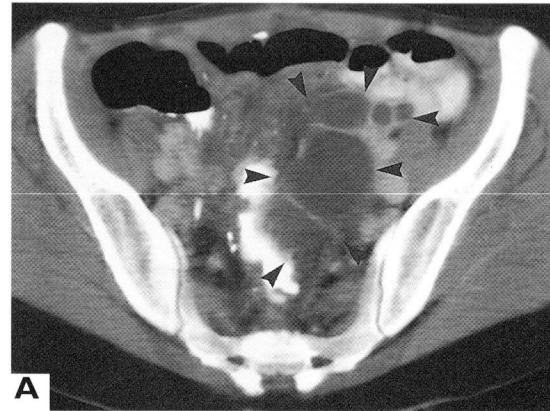

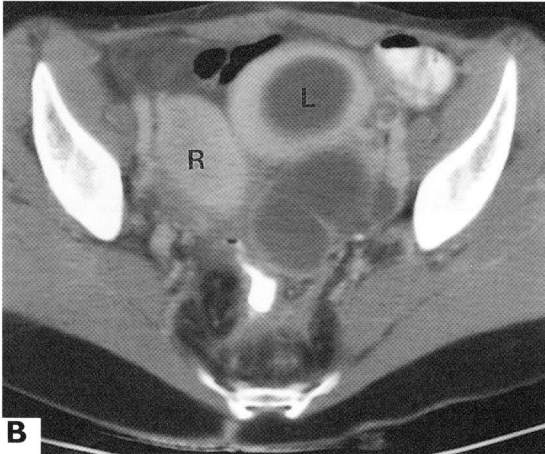

Figure 15.7 Hematosalpinx: (**A**) CT with a fluid-density tubular structure (arrowheads) in the left adnexa. (**B**) This CT, taken 2 cm caudal to A, also shows the tubular structure as well as two uterine cornua (on the right and left). The left horn (L) is distended by low-density material, confirmed at surgery to be a hematosalpinx and hematometra secondary to a unicornuate uterus with a non-communicating left remnant

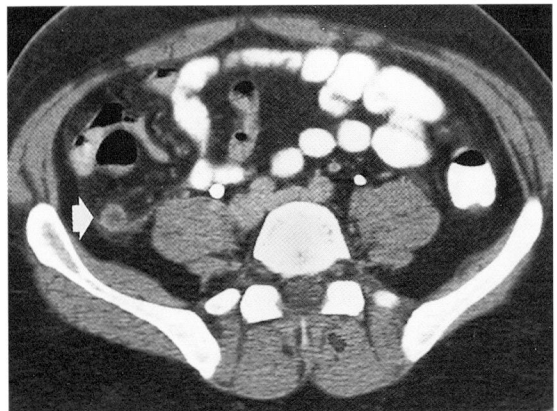

Figure 15.8 Appendicitis: CT showing an enlarged appendix (arrow) with a thickened, abnormally enhanced wall; inflammatory changes can be seen in the adjacent fat. These findings are diagnostic of acute appendicitis

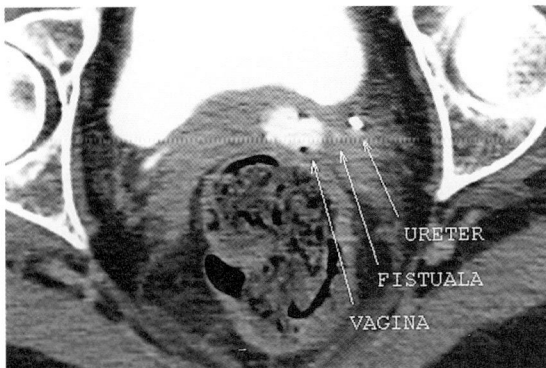

URETER

FISTUALA

VAGINA

Figure 15.9 Postoperative fistula: Posthysterectomy CT in a patient with a suspected urinary fistula to the vagina. A tampon was placed in the vagina and narrow slices were obtained after administration of intravenous contrast. A thin fistula between the left ureter and vagina can be seen

sensitivity in examining the adnexa renders it less helpful in young women than in others, CT should be considered especially when the symptoms have been prolonged and an abscess is likely. The appendix is identified as a tubular structure arising from the cecum and is abnormal if there is wall thickening, enlargement or increased density in the periappendiceal fat[5] (Figure 15.8).

Postoperative studies

The appearance of a postoperative abscess is similar to that of a tuboovarian abscess, although the location is more variable. CT has advantages over ultrasound particularly in identifying intraloop abscesses and when ultrasound is hindered by patient pain and bowel gas associated with postoperative ileus. Fistulas (Figure 15.9) and other abnormalities may also be demonstrated.

Adenopathy

Lymph nodes are identified as well-defined soft tissue-density structures adjacent to the pelvic vasculature. The obturator nodes are particularly important because they are a common site of first spread of many pelvic tumors. Involvement by tumor can be predicted on the basis of size: a short-axis diameter > 15 mm is considered to be abnormal whereas those that are 11–14 mm are considered indeterminate[6].

Ovarian vein thrombosis

Ovarian vein thrombosis can be a difficult diagnosis to confirm. The characteristic CT finding is a well-defined tubular mass extending from the pelvis to the inferior vena cava or left renal vein. This represents enlargement of the ovarian vein with a central area of low density indicating thrombus (Figure 15.10). CT is superior to both ultrasound and MRI in the diagnosis of this condition[7].

Magnetic resonance imaging

Technique

Although a lengthy explanation of the physics of MRI is beyond the scope of this chapter, a brief explanation will allow the

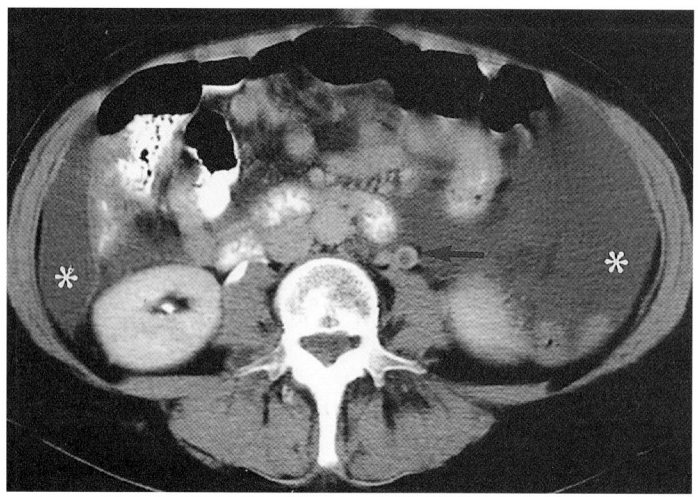

Figure 15.10 Ovarian vein thrombosis: CT taken through the lower abdomen demonstrates a low-density thrombus within the left ovarian vein (arrow) in a patient with recurrent ovarian cancer. Note the ascitic fluid in both paracolic gutters (*)

gynecologist to understand the terminology used to describe the findings with these studies. MRI uses a wide, static, magnetic field to align protons within the body. A short burst of electromagnetic radiation in the radiowave-frequency range is then applied to the patient to disturb the aligned protons from the baseline state. This is followed by the release of electromagnetic radiation from the protons within the patient as they subsequently relax back to the baseline state; it is this radiation that is detected by the MRI unit. The released energy forms the basis of the image and the amount of signal detected is displayed on a gray scale. Regions that give off no signal are black whereas regions that indicate the most signal are white and the intermediate tissues are manifested as appropriate shades of gray.

Differences in the amount of signal emanating from tissues are due to three factors: T_1 relaxation time; T_2 relaxation time; and density of mobile protons. These factors are intrinsic to a tissue and are constant. Variations in the way a particular sequence excites the tissue will change the relative effect that each of these three factors has on the final image. Accordingly, sequences which accentuate the effects of the T_1 relaxation time are referred to as 'T_1-weighted sequences' and those that accentuate the T_2 relaxation time are called 'T_2-weighted sequences'. In evaluating the uterus, T_2-weighted images are the most helpful. In general, however, the signal intensity of a structure as determined on several different sequences is needed to fully characterize the structure.

Gadolinium is attached to a complex molecule (for safety purposes) and used as an intravenous contrast agent similar to the iodinated contrast agents used in CT. Regions enhanced with gadolinium are high in signal (white) on appropriate sequences. In general, gadolinium agents are considerably safer than iodinated agents and are associated with a much lower incidence of allergic reactions and renal complications. There are a number of relative and absolute contraindications to the use of MRI, but these are beyond the scope of this chapter. Most centers screen the patient for these contraindications both at the time of making an appointment and immediately before the study is carried out.

Normal pelvic anatomy on MRI

The uterus is well demonstrated on MRI (Figure 15.11 A and B). As with ultrasonog-

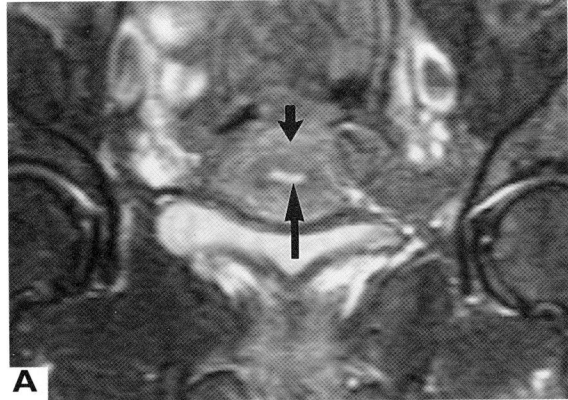

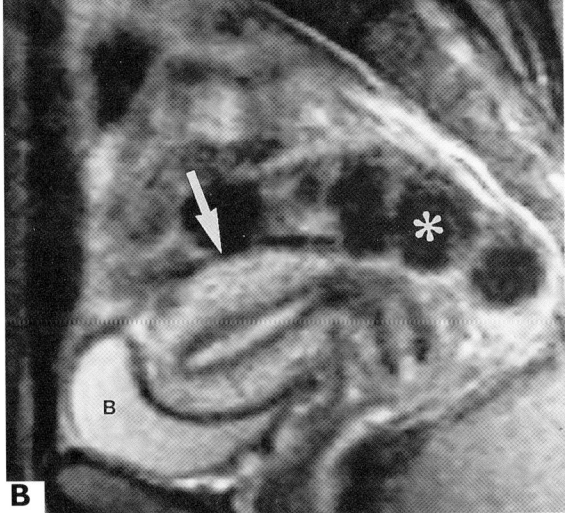

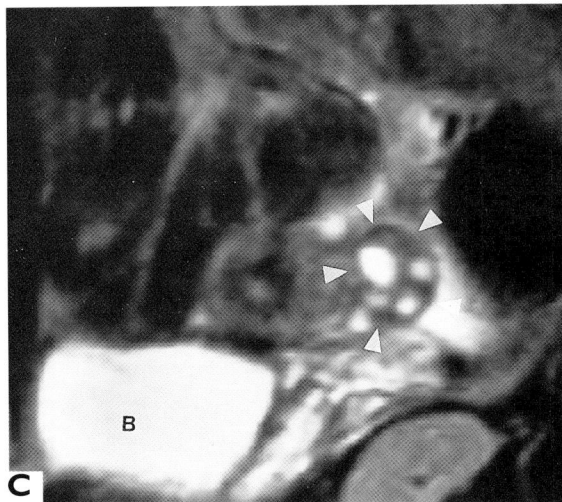

Figure 15.11 Normal MRIs of the pelvis. (**A**) Short-axis T$_2$-weighted MRI of the uterus (nearly coronal to the patient) shows that the myometrium has an intermediate signal intensity (short arrow) and the endometrium (long arrow) has a high signal intensity; the low-signal junctional zone is faintly visualized between the two. (**B**) Sagittal midline MRI reveals an anteflexed uterus (arrow) with normal zonal anatomy. The bladder is anterior and air is seen in the rectosigmoid colon (*). (**C**) Sagittal MRI obtained more laterally (same patient as in B) shows a normal ovary (arrowheads) with several high-signal follicles. B, bladder

raphy, the appearance will vary through the menstrual cycle. The zonal anatomy is best identified on T$_2$-weighted images. The zones or layers identified are the myometrium, junctional zone and endometrium. The signal intensity of the myometrium changes according to the phase of the menstrual cycle, increasing during the secretory phase due to increased fluid content[8]. The middle layer, or junctional zone, has a low signal intensity and represents the longitudinally orientated smooth muscle of the basal layer of the myometrium[9]. The appearance is of a thin low signal-intensity line between the high-signal endometrium and intermediate-signal myometrium (Figure 15.11 A), averaging 5 mm in thickness. This layer does not change during the menstrual cycle, but may become attenuated in the menopause. The endometrium is high in signal on T$_2$-weighted images and becomes progressively thicker through the menstrual cycle. The endometrium is measured on sagittal T$_2$-weighted images through the middle portion of the uterus, including both layers. In premenopausal women, it ranges in thickness from 3–10 mm whereas, in postmenopausal women who are not taking exogenous hormones, it should be no thicker than 4 mm[10].

The cervix is predominantly low in signal intensity on T$_2$-weighted images due to its dense fibrous stroma. Centrally located is a thin high signal-intensity stripe representing the endocervix with glandular fluid and mucus.

The vagina is best visualized on axial T_2-weighted images. An H-shaped high signal-intensity line represents the collapsed mucosa and any fluid or secretions within the vagina. This is surrounded by the intermediate to low signal-intensity muscular wall and the high signal-intensity perivaginal venous plexus. The urethra can be identified as a round structure lying immediately anterior to the vagina and also surrounded by the venous plexus.

The normal ovaries are reliably identified on MRI (Figure 15.11 C). They are usually most easily found on T_2-weighted sequences as oval-shaped structures with multiple, small, high signal-intensity follicles.

Indications for pelvic MRI

The routine use of MRI to evaluate disease of the female pelvis has been limited despite the fact that there are several conditions that are

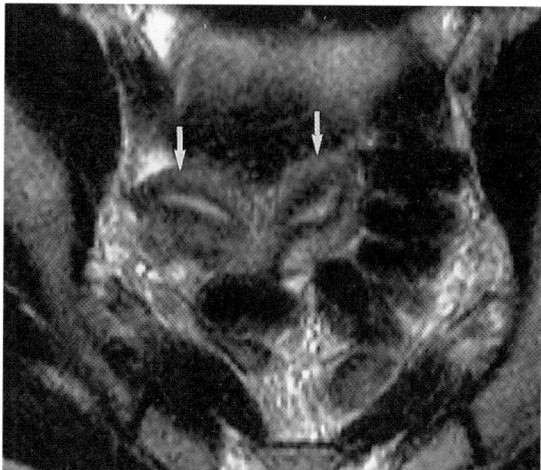

Figure 15.12 Congenital anomaly: Axial T_2-weighted MRI shows a patient with a bicornuate uterus (both horns are arrowed). A scan through the abdomen identified agenesis of the left kidney (not shown here)

better demonstrated by MRI than any other imaging modality. These conditions include congenital uterine anomalies, leiomyomas and adenomyosis. Limited access, perceived cost differentials and lack of physician awareness may account for some of the underuse of MRI[11]. Indeed, there is some evidence that the use of MRI may decrease medical costs. Schwartz and colleagues[12] have examined the impact of MRI studies of the female pelvis on treatment decisions and net cost of treatment. Their results demonstrated that treatment plans after the use of MRI included fewer operations and an increased use of less invasive surgery, representing overall savings in the treatment of the 69 women in their sample.

Findings on pelvic MRI

Uterus

Congenital anomalies

MRI is an excellent modality for demonstrating the full spectrum of congenital uterine anomalies. The multiplanar ability of MRI allows the routine display of coronal long-axis images of the uterus. MRI provides excellent visualization of both the endometrium and myometrium to combine, in one study, the advantages of both hysterosalpingography and ultrasonography. In a study of 26 patients with Müllerian duct anomalies, MRI was 100% accurate in the diagnoses, whereas ultrasound was 92% accurate and hysterosalpingography only 16% accurate[13]. Of particular value is the accuracy of MRI in differentiating a septate uterus which can be treated through the hysteroscope from the bicornuate uterus which cannot (Figure 15.12). MRI alone may be able to provide an accurate and adequate preoperative assessment in patients with uterine and vaginal septa[14] (Figure 15.13).

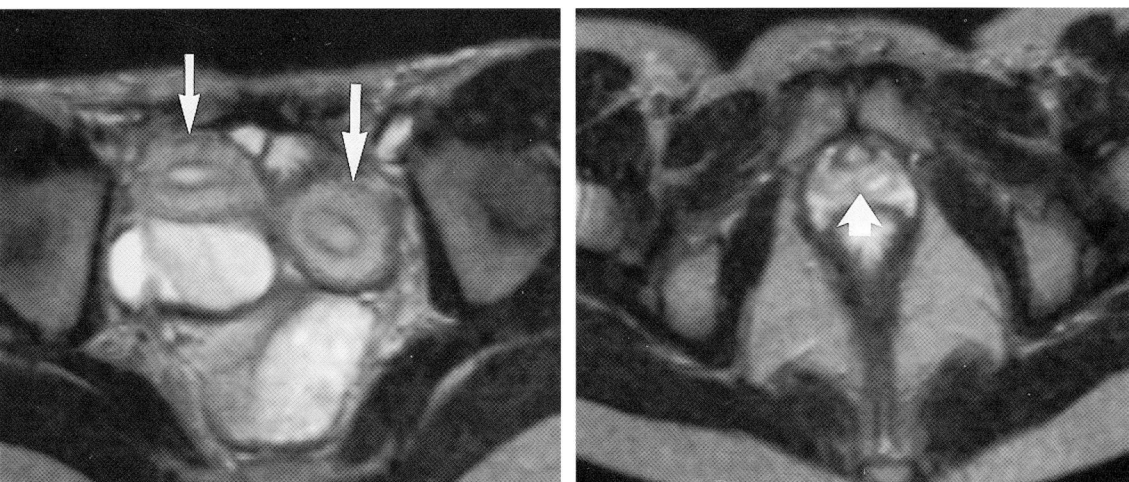

Figure 15.13 Congenital anomaly: Two MRIs taken through the pelvis of a patient with a didelphic uterus show the two uterine horns (arrowed; left) and a septate vagina (arrowed; right)

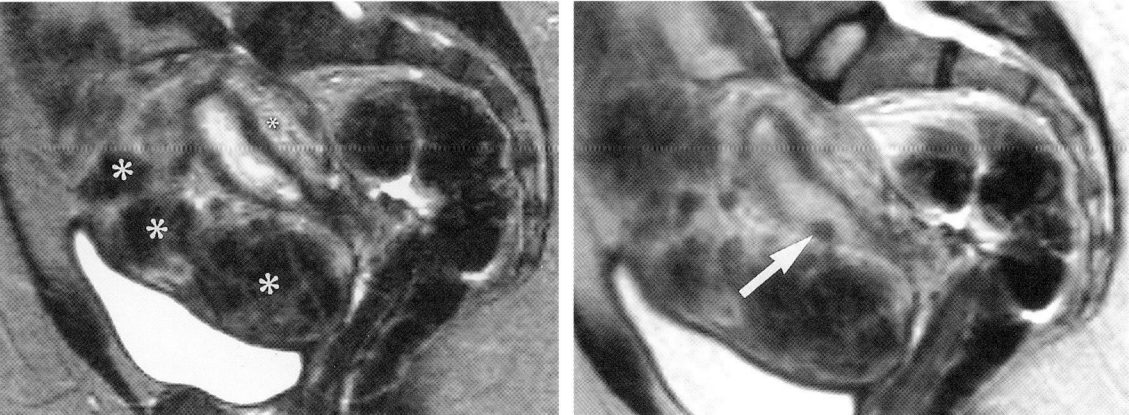

Figure 15.14 Leiomyomas: Sagittal midline MRI (left) showing the zonal anatomy of the uterus and multiple hypointense intramural uterine leiomyomas (*) predominantly in the anterior wall of the uterus. Note the relatively high signal of the myometrium, which is consistent with the secretory phase of the menstrual cycle. Adjacent image (right; same patient) shows a 5-mm submucous leiomyoma (arrowed)

Leiomyoma

Leiomyomas usually appear as well-defined, homogeneous, low signal-intensity uterine masses on T_2-weighted images[15]. Use of imaging planes in both the short and long axis of the uterus provides sufficient information to assign specific locations as well as to differentiate submucous, intramural and subserosal tumors (Figure 15.14). MRI has been demonstrated to be more accurate than ultrasonography in diagnosing leiomyomas and in correct assessment of uterine location[16,17] (Figure 15.15). This is especially helpful in preoperative planning. Also, MRI readily differentiates pedunculated submucosal leiomyomas from other solid pelvic masses when ultrasound is indeterminate[18].

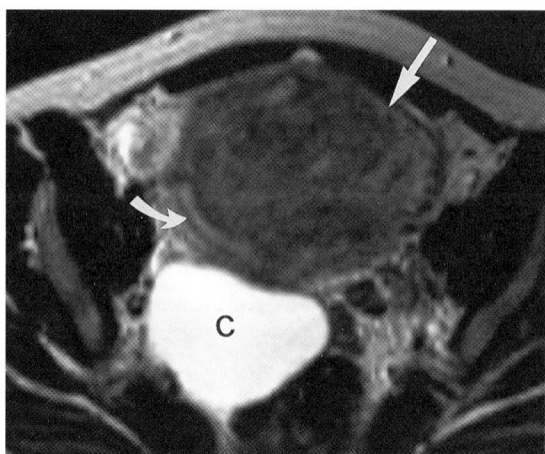

Figure 15.15 Leiomyoma: A single-axial MRI shows a large low signal-intensity anterior intramural leiomyoma (arrow). The endometrium (curved arrow) is well visualized whereas it was not identified on ultrasound. Also seen is a high signal-intensity ovarian cyst (C)

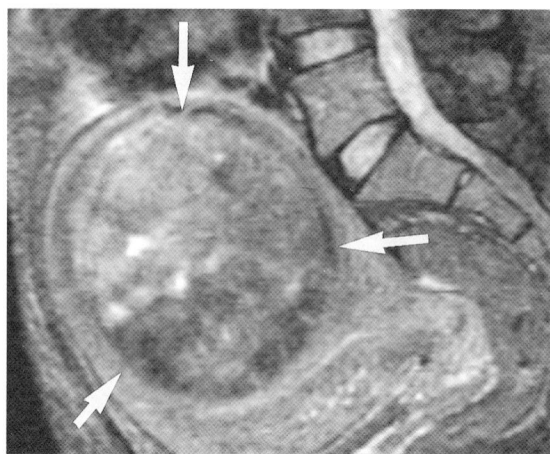

Figure 15.16 Degenerate leiomyoma: Sagittal T_2-weighted MRI shows a large posterior intramural leiomyoma (arrowed) containing areas of low and high signal. The high-signal areas may also represent cellularity

Complications within leiomyomas are also identified by MRI. A minority of leiomyomas have areas of high signal intensity on T_2-weighted images which may represent either degeneration or cellularity[19] (Figure 15.16). Dynamic gadolinium administration may differentiate the two conditions; this has prognostic value as cellular leiomyomas can be significantly reduced in size following treatment with gonadotropin-releasing hormone (Gn-RH) analogues whereas degenerated leiomyomas cannot[19]. Red degeneration of a leiomyoma may have the specific appearance of a hyperintense rim on T_1-weighted images which is, however, hypointense on T_2-weighted images[20] (see Figure 15.21); this may prove useful in the evaluation of symptomatic patients. As with ultrasound and CT, MRI cannot identify sarcomatous degeneration within a leiomyoma.

Adenomyosis

Adenomyosis can be difficult to diagnose clinically, ultrasonographically and inva-

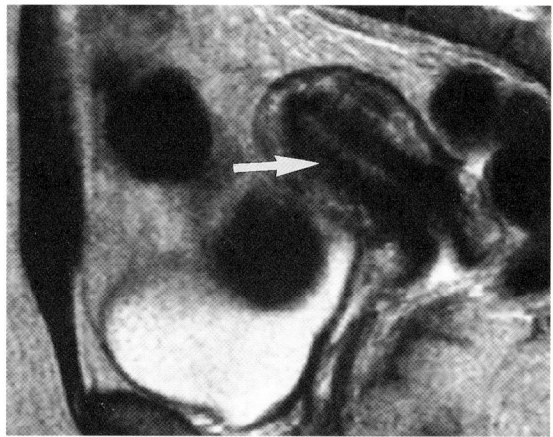

Figure 15.17 Adenomyosis: Sagittal T_2-weighted MRI shows an abnormally thickened junctional zone (arrow) which is consistent with adenomyosis

sively. MRI has been shown to be superior to endovaginal ultrasound in the diagnosis of adenomyosis[21] (Figure 15.17). Diffuse or focal thickening of the junctional zone of >5 mm is the most common finding in adenomyosis. Occasionally, high signal-intensity regions in the junctional or myo-

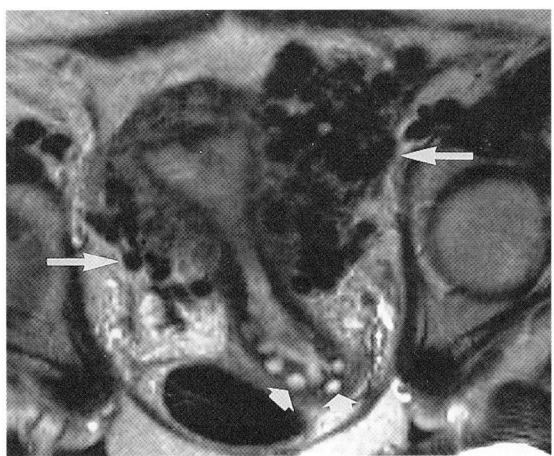

Figure 15.18 Uterine arteriovenous malformation: Oblique coronal T_2-weighted MRI (in long axis of uterus) shows bilateral serpiginous vessels in the myometrium and adjacent parametrium (arrows), which appear black due to the blood flowing within them. Note the multiple nabothian cysts within the cervix (short arrow)

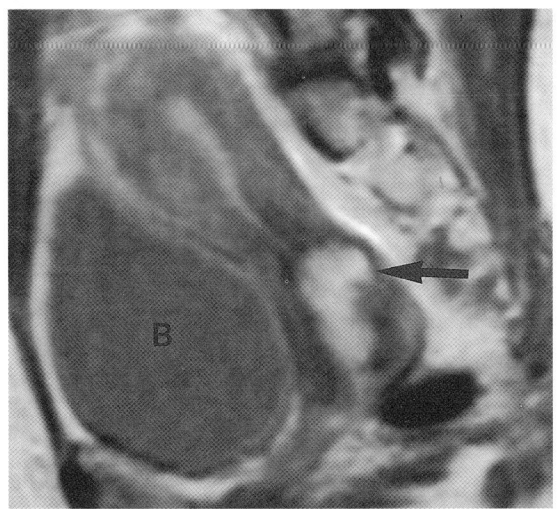

Figure 15.19 Cervical carcinoma: Sagittal MRI showing a lobulated high signal-intensity mass (arrow) distending the cervix, but not extending beyond the cervical stroma. The bladder (B) is seen anteriorly

metrial zones can also be identified. Particularly helpful is the differentiation between adenomyosis and leiomyomas in patients presenting with an enlarged uterus. Togashi

and colleagues[22] examined 93 women with uterine enlargement prospectively; of the 71 who had leiomyomas and the 16 with adenomyosis, all but one were correctly diagnosed by MRI.

Vascular malformation

These are easily identified on MRI due to the flow of blood within the vessels which can be identified on many sequences as an absent signal (Figure 15.18). MRI can be used for preoperative or preembolization planning.

Cervix

Cervical carcinoma

The potential role of MRI is not in the diagnosis of cervical carcinoma, but rather in the improvement of its staging (Figure 15.19). There is at present no general acceptance of a role for MRI in this process, although several centers are endeavoring to improve the accuracy of MRI with the use of new techniques.

Nabothian cysts

Although there is no need to diagnose these cysts by MRI, they are a common finding and should not be confused with other lesions. These cysts are identified as well-defined round cervical masses that are isointense on T_1-weighted images and high in signal intensity on T_2-weighted images[23] (Figure 15.20).

Endometrium

Endometrial carcinoma

Although abnormalities of the endometrium are demonstrated by MRI, the findings are non-specific. Early endometrial carcinoma and endometrial hyperplasia have a similar appearance (endometrial thickness > 4 mm in

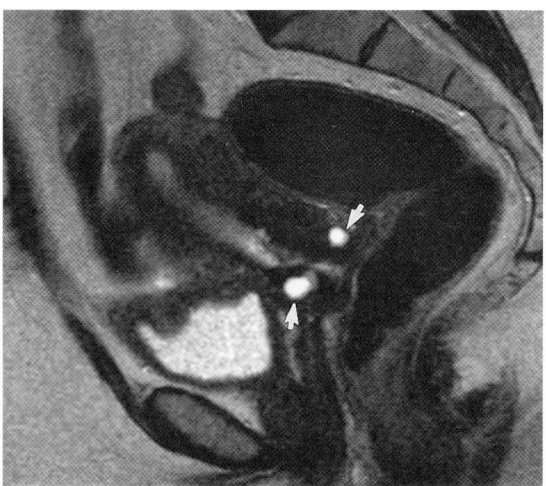

Figure 15.20 Nabothian cysts: Sagittal T_2-weighted MRI through the uterus and cervix showing two well-defined, high signal-intensity, round nabothian cysts (arrows) in the cervix

postmenopausal women), and a histological diagnosis is required[24]. MRI has been successfully used in some centers to predict the invasion of myometrium and for local staging in cases of known endometrial carcinoma[25]. Loss of the junctional zone can be predictive of invasion into the under-lying myometrium; MRI is 85% accurate in predicting the depth of such invasion[26].

Endometrial polyp

In one study[27], the detection of endometrial polyps was found to be 79% with MRI. However, benign polyps cannot be reliably distinguished from polypoid endometrial cancer. Submucous leiomyomas are differentiated by their characteristic low signal intensity on T_2-weighted images.

Adnexa

Adnexal cystic mass

Adnexal masses are identified on MRI with a 95% sensitivity[28] (Figure 15.21; see also

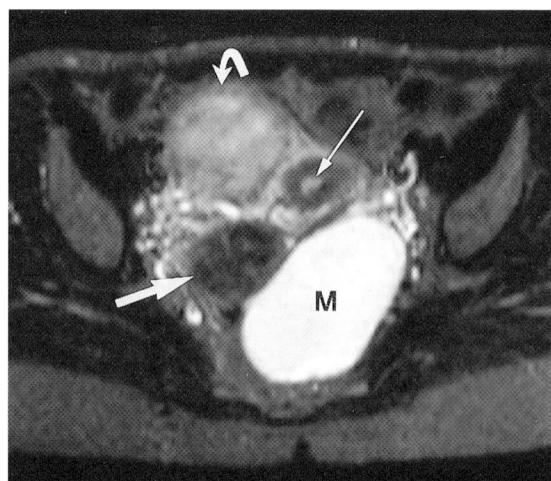

Figure 15.21 Mucinous cystadenocarcinoma: T_2-weighted MRI (short-axis plane through the uterus) demonstrates the high-signal endometrium (thin arrow) surrounded by the junctional zone. Also seen are a hypointense subserosal leiomyoma (arrow), a high-signal subserosal degenerating leiomyoma (curved arrow) and a left-sided cystic adnexal mass (M) which proved to be a mucinous cystadenocarcinoma

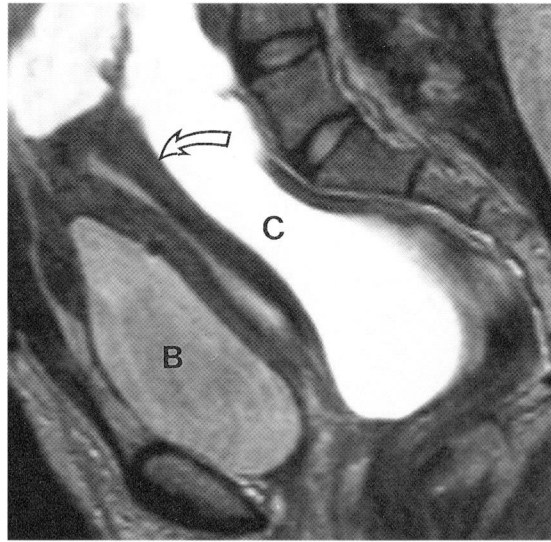

Figure 15.22 Peritoneal inclusion cyst: T_2-weighted MRI shows a high signal-intensity oblong cyst (C) displacing the uterus (arrow) anteriorly which proved, at surgery, to represent a peritoneal inclusion cyst. The bladder (B) is seen anteriorly

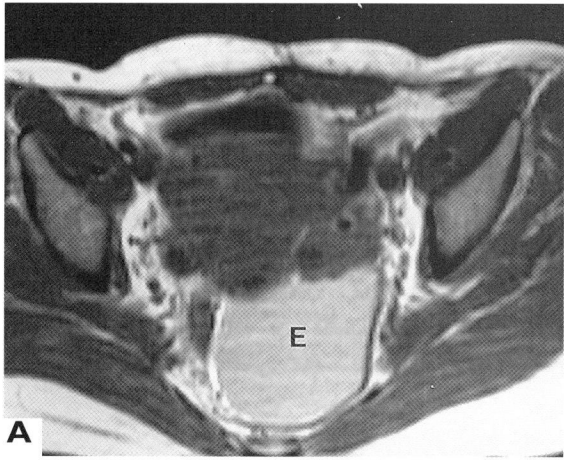

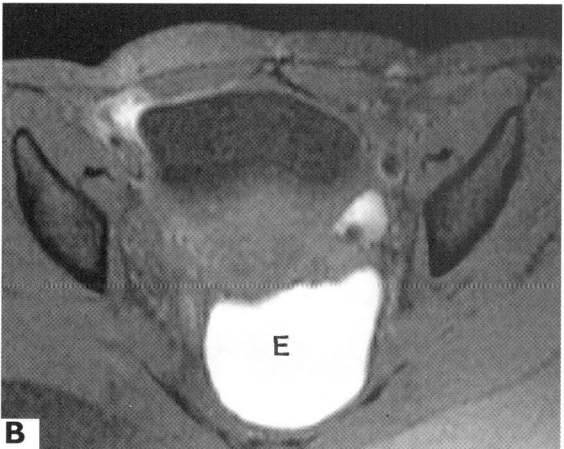

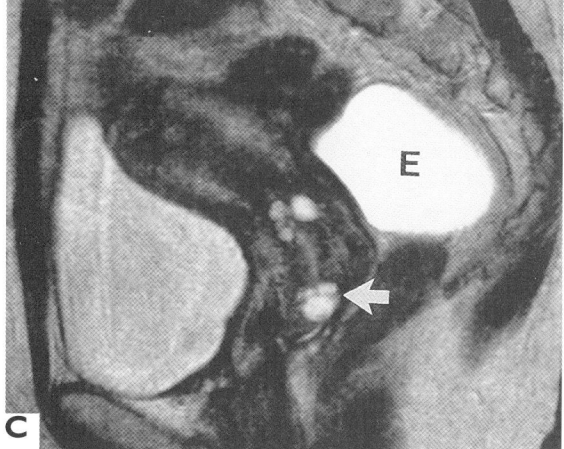

Figure 15.23 Endometrioma. (**A**) Axial T_1-weighted MRI shows a well-defined mass (E) with high signal intensity posterior to the uterus. The mass could represent fat in a cystic teratoma or hemorrhage in an endometrioma. (**B**) Chemically selective fat-saturated T_1-weighted MRI shows the mass (E) to remain high in signal intensity whereas the fat in the bone marrow and subcutaneous tissues has been suppressed, indicating that the lesion is an endometrioma. (**C**) Sagittal T_2-weighted MRI shows the endometrioma (E) to be high-signal; multiple nabothian cysts are also present (arrow)

Figure 15.15). However, the appearance of many adnexal masses is non-specific and, as with ultrasound, malignant masses cannot be completely distinguished from benign. However, several entities, including dermoid cysts, most endometriomas, pedunculated leiomyomas, hydrosalpinx and ovarian fibromas, can have specific findings and be characterized by MRI[11]. Follicular, corpus luteal and simple cysts all appear as high-signal, homogeneous, well-defined masses with no identifiable wall (Figure 15.22). Ovarian carcinomas tend to be larger with demonstrable solid components.

Endometrioma

Endometriomas typically appear as round or oval well-defined adnexal masses with a thick low-signal wall and a central high signal on T_1-weighted sequences (Figures 15.23 A and C). When this pattern is found, MRI is between 91% and 98% specific in making the diagnosis[11]. Lipid within a cystic teratoma may have a similar appearance on standard sequences; for this reason, special fat-suppression sequences are used to differentiate these lesions[29] (Figure 15.23 B).

Cystic teratoma (dermoid)

Using standard as well as fat-suppressing imaging sequences, lipid can be identified with confidence. The presence of lipid in an adnexal mass identifies it, for practical purposes, as a dermoid; MRI is highly specific in making this diagnosis[11].

Conclusions

Although other methods of evaluating the female pelvis, including laparoscopy, hysteroscopy, colposcopy and ultrasonography, are often superior in both sensitivity and specificity to either CT or MRI, it is still incumbent on the gynecologist to understand these techniques. There are a few indications in which CT and MRI are superior to other modalities. The global view provided by these modalities can be very helpful in many confusing clinical settings. Furthermore, many patients undergo these studies for other reasons and are subsequently referred to the gynecologist because of the abnormalities of the female genital tract which are revealed. Understanding the value and limitations of the initial modality will enable the practitioner to proceed logically with further studies or treatment.

References

1. Casillas J, Joseph RC, Guerra JJ. CT appearance of uterine leiomyomas. *Radiographics* 1990;10:999–1007

2. Buy JN, Ghossain MA, Moss AA, *et al.* Cystic teratoma of the ovary: CT detection. *Radiology* 1989;171:697–701

3. Fukuda T, Ikeuchi M, Hashimoto H, *et al.* Computed tomography of ovarian masses. *J Comput Assist Tomogr* 1986;10:990–6

4. Wilbur AC, Aizenstein RI, Napp TE. CT findings in tuboovarian abscess. *AJR* 1992; 158:575–9

5. Balthazar EJ, Birnbaum BA, Yee J, *et al.* Acute appendicitis: CT and US correlation in 100 patients. *Radiology* 1994;190:31–5

6. Einstein DM, Singer AA, Chilcote WA, Desai RK. Abdominal lymphadenopathy: Spectrum of CT findings. *Radiographics* 1991; 11:457–72

7. Savader SJ, Otero RR, Savader BL. Puerperal ovarian vein thrombosis: Evaluation with CT, US and MR imaging. *Radiology* 1988;167: 637–9

8. McCarthy S, Taubert C, Gore J. Female pelvic anatomy: MR assessment of variations during the menstrual cycle and with use of oral contraceptives. *Radiology* 1986;160:119–23

9. Brown HK, Stoll BS, Nicosia SV, *et al.* Uterine junctional zone: Correlation of histological findings and MR imaging. *Radiology* 1991;179: 409–13

10. Olson M, Posniak H, Tempany CM, Dudiak CM. MR imaging of the female pelvic region. *Radiographics* 1992;12:445–65

11. Outwater EK, Dunton CJ. Imaging of the ovary and adnexa: Clinical issues and applications of MR imaging. *Radiology* 1995;194: 1–18

12. Schwartz LB, Panagaes E, Lange R, *et al.* Female pelvis: Impact of MR imaging on treatment decisions and net cost analysis. *Radiology* 1994;192:55–60

13. Pellerito JS, McCarthy SM, Doyle MB, et al. Diagnosis of uterine anomalies: Relative accuracy of MR imaging, endovaginal sonography and hysterosalpingography. *Radiology* 1992;183:795–800

14. Doyle MB. Magnetic resonance imaging in müllerian fusion defects. *J Reprod Med* 1992;37:33–8

15. Hricak H, Tscholakoff D, Heinrichs L, et al. Uterine leiomyomas: Correlation of MR, histopathologic findings and symptoms. *Radiology* 1986;158:385–91

16. Dudiak CM, Turner DA, Patel SK, et al. Uterine leiomyomas in the infertile patient: Preoperative localization with MR imaging versus US and hysterosalpingography. *Radiology* 1988;167:627–30

17. Riccio TJ, Adams HG, Munzing DE, Mattrey RF. Magnetic resonance imaging as an adjunct to sonography in the evaluation of the female pelvis. *Magn Reson Imaging* 1990;8(6):699–704

18. Weinreb JC, Barkoff ND, Megibow A, Demopoulos R. The value of MR imaging in distinguishing leiomyomas from other solid pelvic masses when sonography is indeterminate. *AJR* 1990;154:295–9

19. Yamashita Y, Torashima M, Takahashi M, et al. Hyperintense uterine leiomyoma at T2-weighted MR imaging: Differentiation with dynamic enhanced MR imaging and clinical implications. *Radiology* 1993;189:721–5

20. Kawakami S, Togashi K, Konishi I, et al. Red degeneration of uterine leiomyoma: MR appearance. *J Comput Assist Tomogr* 1994;18(6):925–8

21. Ascher SM, Arnold LL, Patt RH, et al. Adenomyosis: Prospective comparison of MR imaging and transvaginal sonography. *Radiology* 1994;190:803–6

22. Togashi K, Ozasa I, Konishi I, et al. Enlarged uterus: Differentiation between adenomyosis and leiomyoma with MR imaging. *Radiology* 1989;171:531–4

23. Kier R. Nonovarian gynecologic cysts: MR imaging findings. *AJR* 1992;158:1265–9

24. Brown JJ, Thurnher S, Hricak H. MR imaging of the uterus: Low-signal-intensity abnormalities of the endometrium and endometrial cavity. *Magn Reson Imaging* 1990;8(3):309–13

25. Posniak HV, Olson MC. Malignant diseases of the uterus. In Tempany CMC, ed. *MR and Imaging of the Female Pelvis*. St Louis: Mosby, 1995:155–84

26. Yamashita Y, Harada M, Sawada T, et al. Normal uterus and FIGO stage I endometrial carcinoma: Dynamic gadolinium-enhanced MR imaging. *Radiology* 1993;186:495–501

27. Hricak H, Finck S, Honda G, Goranson H. MR imaging in the evaluation of benign uterine masses: Value of gadopentetate dimeglumine-enhanced T1-weighted images. *AJR* 1992;158:1043–50

28. Stevens SK, Hricak H, Stern JL. Ovarian lesions: Detection and characterization with gadolinium-enhanced MR imaging at 1.5T. *Radiology* 1991;181:481–8

29. Stevens SK, Hricak H, Campos Z. Teratomas versus cystic hemorrhagic adnexal lesions: Differentiation with proton-selective fat-saturation MR imaging. *Radiology* 1993;186:481–8

16 Uterine pathology

Debra S. Heller

The pathology laboratory often receives specimens obtained during hysteroscopy and is able to confirm the hysteroscopic impression. Although many of these specimens are identical in appearance to those obtained by other operative modalities, some specimens are received in fragments or with cautery artifact after operative hysteroscopic resection, thereby occasionally hampering interpretation. The various types of specimens received by the pathology laboratory from hysteroscopic procedures are listed in Table 16.1.

Abnormal uterine bleeding

Abnormal uterine bleeding may occur under a variety of conditions. After eliminating non-uterine causes such as systemic disease or non-genital bleeding, and ruling out pregnancy-related bleeding, uterine bleeding may be classified as either organic or dysfunctional. Organic causes of bleeding are those associated with intrinsic uterine pathology, such as a polyp or submucous leiomyoma. Dysfunctional uterine bleeding (DUB) is secondary to an imbalance of the hormonal milieu. The endometrium in cases of DUB may appear completely normal or may show a variety of patterns, both non-secretory and secretory.

Menstrual cycle

Endometrial samples obtained during an infertility work-up as well as in some cases of dysfunctional bleeding may be completely

Table 16.1 Pathology specimens from hysteroscopic procedures

Endometrium
  history of abnormal bleeding
  infertility work-up
  abnormal transvaginal ultrasound
  abnormal Papanicolaou smear
  follow-up after hyperplasia
  endometrial polyps
  endometrial carcinoma
Retained IUD / foreign bodies
Retained products of conception / placental polyps
Endocervical polyps
Uterine septa / synechiae
Submucous smooth muscle neoplasms
Adenomyosis

normal on histology. In these cases, the clinical history is important in determining whether the specimen is out of phase. Luteal phase defects, defined as a >2-day discrepancy in clinical and histological dating may be seen in some cases of infertility and DUB, but also occur in completely asymptomatic fertile women.

During the first half of the menstrual cycle, under the stimulus of estrogen, the endometrium becomes taller, with increased gland complexity and mitotic activity. Proliferative endometrium cannot be dated, but can be divided into early, mid- and late proliferative phases by the morphology. Early proliferative endometrium (cycle days 1–4) is characterized by simple straight glands, which appear small and round on histological section. Mitotic activity is present in both glands and stroma (Figure 16.1).

During the midproliferative phase (cycle days 5–9), gland complexity and mitotic activity both increase, the endometrium becomes taller and stromal edema may be seen (Figure 16.2). Late proliferative endometrium (cycle days 10–14) is taller than early and midproliferative endometrium, and shows maximum mitotic activity. The glands are more complex in architecture, and the edema seen in the midproliferative phase is absent (Figure 16.3). In all phases of proliferative endometrium, the glandular epithelium is pseudostratified, thereby distinguishing it from the single layer of secretory endometrium.

Secretory endometrium can be reliably dated on a daily basis, as first described by Noyes and colleagues[1]. Secretory endometrium can also be divided into early (cycle days 15–19), mid (cycle days 20–24) and late (cycle days 25–28). It was originally thought that, whereas the proliferative phase of the cycle was variable, the secretory phase was fixed at 14 days. This has proved to be not the case and normally fertile women can have variable cycles[2]. For this reason, it is better not to diagnose a luteal phase defect unless the endometrium is more than 2 days out of phase in more than one cycle.

During the early secretory phase, it is not possible to determine histologically whether or not ovulation has occurred until cycle day 17. Day 15 endometrium may show a few subnuclear vacuoles and up to 50% of

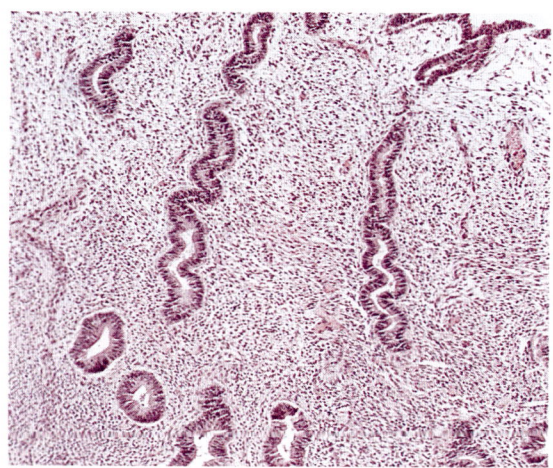

Figure 16.2 Midproliferative endometrium shows increased gland complexity and an edematous stroma (H & E)

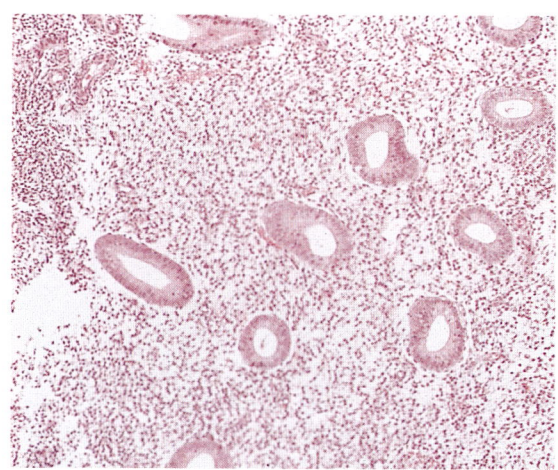

Figure 16.1 Early proliferative endometrium showing small tubular glands. Glandular epithelium is pseudostratified and mitotically active (H & E)

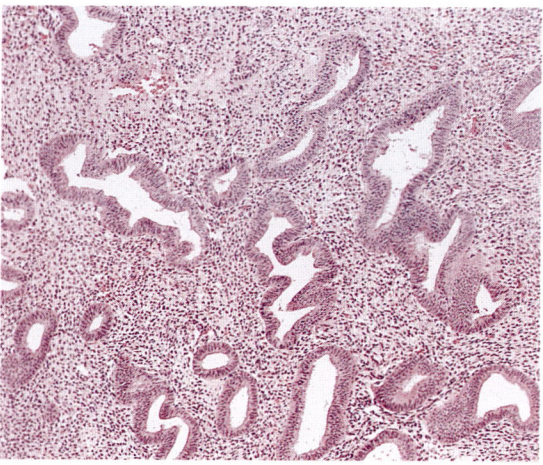

Figure 16.3 Late proliferative endometrium showing markedly increased gland tortuosity. Peak glandular and stromal mitotic activity occurs at this time (H & E)

glands may show subnuclear vacuolization on day 16, but this may be seen secondary to estrogenic stimulation alone in the absence of progesterone; mitotic activity is still abundant. The morphology of day 17 endometrium (Figure 16.4) allows a reliable determination that ovulation has occurred. The glands show uniform subnuclear vacuolization and give the appearance of piano keys. At day 17, there is only a single layer of glandular epithelium and mitotic activity is minimal. As the early secretory phase progresses, the vacuoles migrate to a supranuclear location, with peak secretion on day 20. It is often difficult to assign an exact day to endometrium in the day 19–21 range (Figure 16.5), but peak stromal edema is seen on day 22 (Figure 16.6) and spiral arterioles become prominent on day 23 (Figure 16.7). Predecidual cuffing is present around the spiral arterioles and spreads outwards during the late secretory period. There is increased cuffing on day 24, the presence of predecidua under the surface by day 25 and complete stromal predecidualization by day 27 (Figure 16.8). Breakdown and menses begin on day 28. Menstrual endometrium is characterized by gland-stroma dissociation,

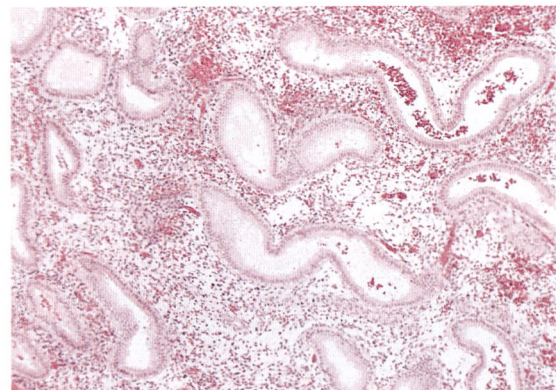

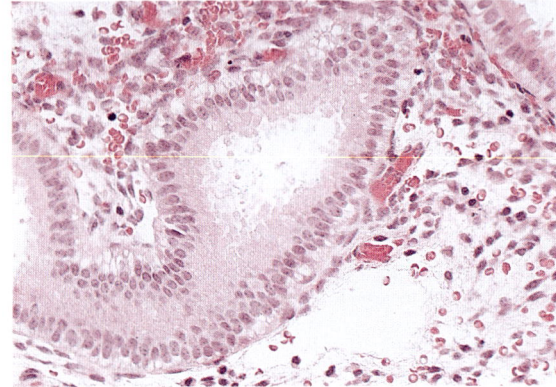

Figure 16.5 Day 19–21 secretory endometrium in low- (upper) and high- (lower) power views showing both subnuclear and supranuclear vacuoles. The glandular epithelium is single-layered and lacks mitotic activity (H & E)

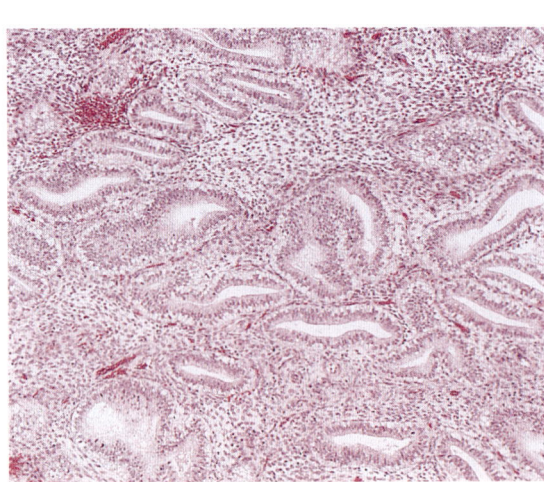

Figure 16.4 Day 17 secretory endometrium showing uniform subnuclear vacuoles (H & E)

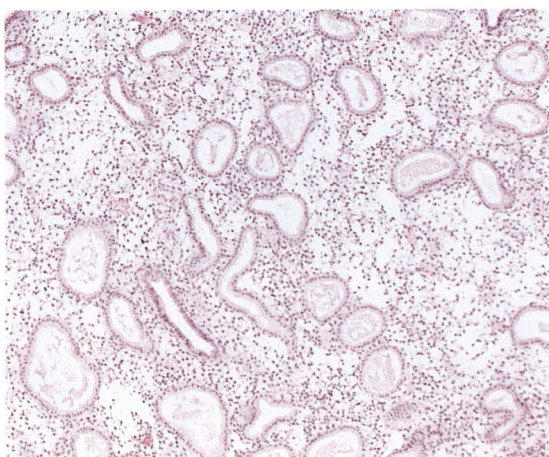

Figure 16.6 Day 22 secretory endometrium shows peak stromal edema (H & E)

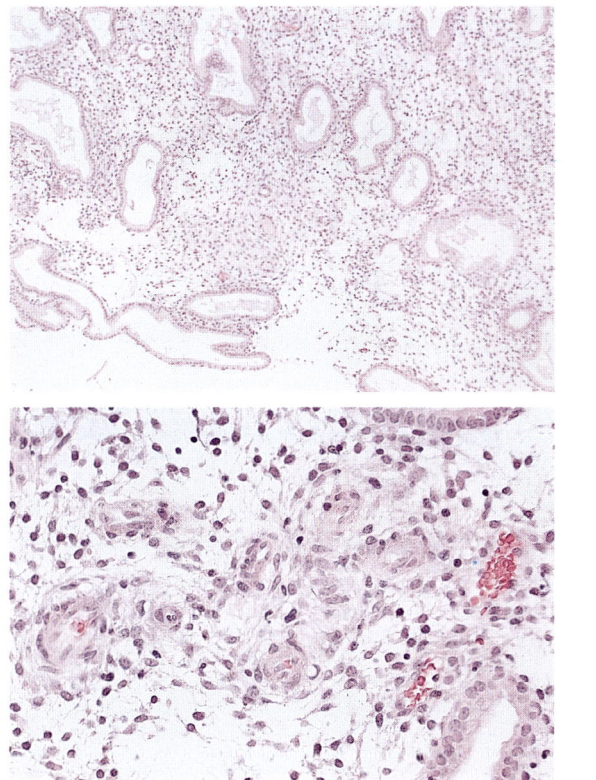

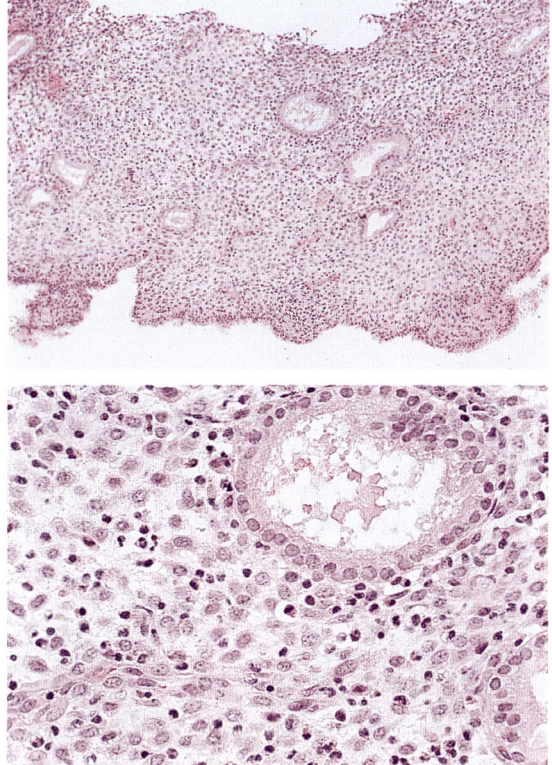

Figure 16.7 Day 23 secretory endometrium in low- (upper) and high- (lower) power views shows prominent spiral arterioles with perivascular cuffing by predecidua (H & E)

Figure 16.8 Low- (upper) and high- (lower) power views of day 27 secretory endometrium show complete predecidualization of the stroma (H & E)

stromal clumping, fibrin thrombi in vessels and nuclear 'dust' (Figure 16.9).

Atrophy

Postmenopausal endometrium may exhibit one of two common atrophic patterns: atrophy may be diffuse, with a thin endometrium and inactive glands (Figure 16.10); or it may occur in another common pattern, cystic atrophy, with widely dilated glands (Figure 16.11). This latter pattern may be distinguished from hyperplasia by the flat epithelium in the cystic glands, which are devoid of mitotic activity.

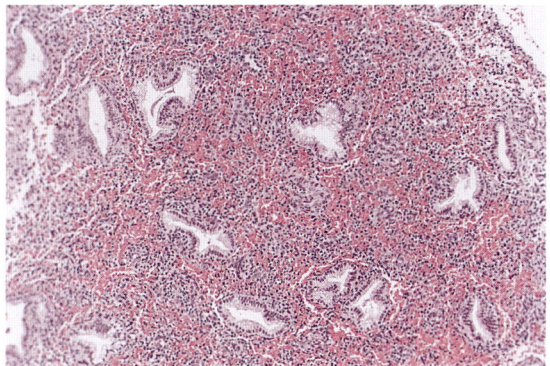

Figure 16.9 Menstrual endometrium shows breakdown and stromal clumping. Only from early menstrual endometrium is it possible to determine whether ovulation has occurred. In this example, secretory changes are still recognizable (H & E)

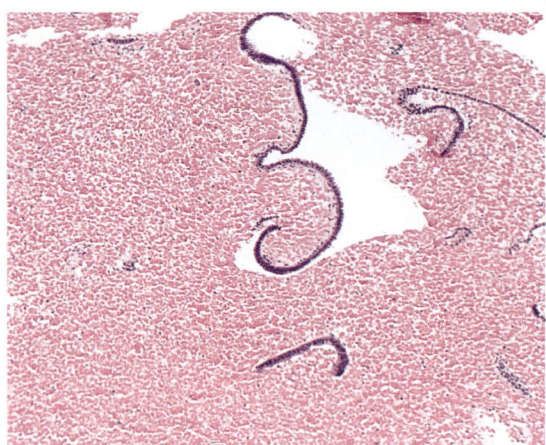

Figure 16.10 Atrophied endometrium is often seen in specimens from postmenopausal women; only superficial strips of inactive glandular epithelium are seen here (H & E)

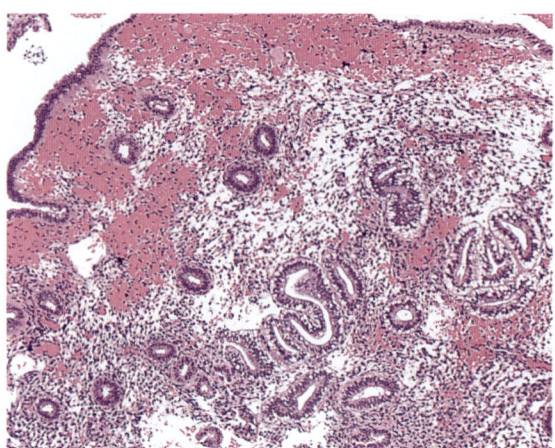

Figure 16.12 Hormone replacement therapy can result in an endometrium showing both proliferative and secretory features, as seen here (H & E)

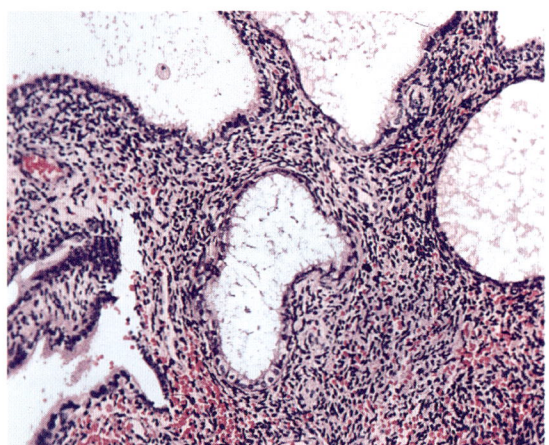

Figure 16.11 Cystic atrophy is characterized by cystically dilated glands lined by flattened inactive epithelium (H & E)

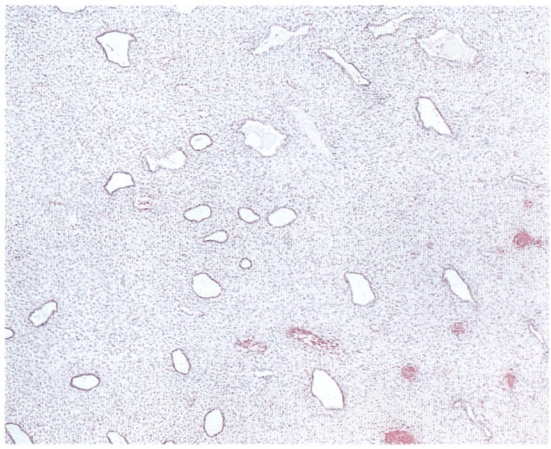

Figure 16.13 Progesterone therapy can result in a picture of inactive glands in a decidualized stroma (H & E)

Iatrogenic hormonal effects

Endometrium stimulated by exogenous hormone therapy shows a pattern that reflects both the medication, dose and duration as well as the underlying hormonal milieu of the patient. This is particularly evident in postmenopausal women receiving estrogen / progesterone replacement therapy, when the endometrium may appear atrophic, proliferative, secretory or irregular, with mixed proliferative and secretory features (Figure 16.12). If estrogen stimulation is excessive, hyperplastic and malignant patterns may also be seen.

Prolonged oral contraception as well as progestational therapy for abnormal bleeding results in endometrium with small atrophic glands and decidualized stroma (Figure 16.13). Therapy with gonadotropin-

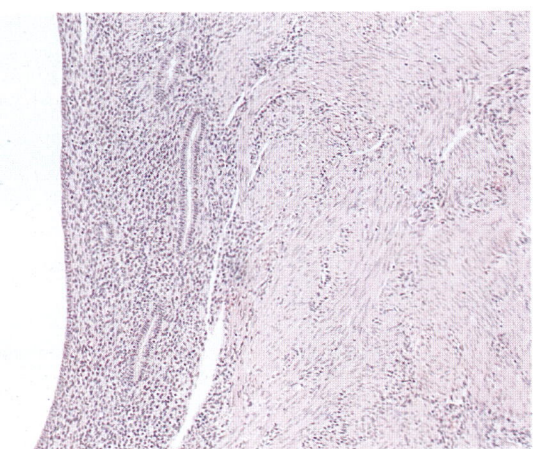

Figure 16.14 Gn-RH agonist therapy may result in an atrophic endometrium (H & E)

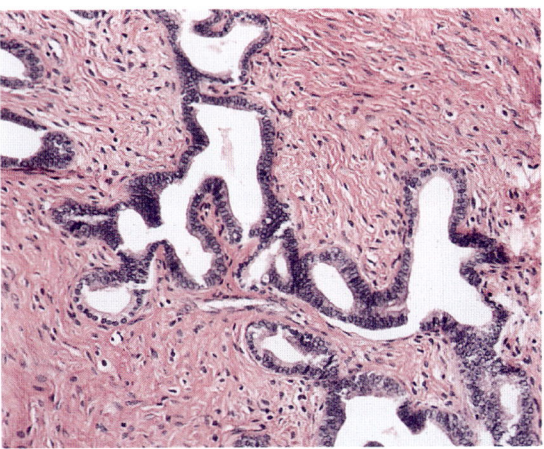

Figure 16.15 Endometrial polyps from patients taking tamoxifen are often large, with cystically dilated glands and a densely fibrous stroma (H & E)

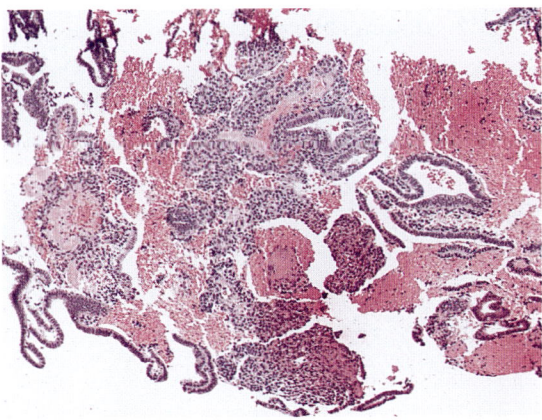

Figure 16.16 Anovulatory menstrual endometrium exhibiting breakdown on a background of disordered proliferation (see Figure 16.17; H & E)

releasing hormone (Gn-RH) agonists creates an artificial menopause with an atrophic endometrium (Figure 16.14). Tamoxifen, which exerts an antiestrogenic effect on breast carcinoma, has a weak estrogenic effect on the postmenopausal uterus. In addition to endometrial hyperplasia and carcinoma, endometrial and endocervical polyps, and growth of adenomyosis, endometriosis and leiomyomas have been described. Endometrial polyps arising after tamoxifen therapy are often large with a densely fibrotic stroma and cystically dilated glands[3] (Figure 16.15).

Dysfunctional uterine bleeding

Dysfunctional uterine bleeding (DUB), defined as bleeding in the absence of systemic disease, pregnancy or intrauterine lesion, is due to hormonal imbalance. Both non-secretory and secretory patterns may be seen[4]. The most common cause of DUB is anovulation. Anovulatory endometrium may appear as normal proliferative, proliferative with breakdown (Figure 16.16), disordered proliferative or even as hyper-

plasia / carcinoma in the presence of continued unopposed estrogen stimulation. Disordered proliferation (Figure 16.17) is characterized by scattered, cystically dilated, glands in a proliferative background with no increase in the gland : stroma ratio, and is not considered hyperplastic. Endometrial ablation may be performed in cases of recurrent DUB, but does not result in a specimen for pathological evaluation. A more recent technique, endomyometrial resection[5], removes the entire endometrium in strips with myometrium (Figure 16.18).

Endometrial polyps

The ideal endometrial polyp, from a pathologist's point of view, is intact with an endometrial glandular epithelium lining on three sides, and a prominent stalk with thick-walled vessels. Often, polyps are removed in fragments, and the irregular, stellate, non-secretory glands and fibrotic stroma have to be relied upon to make the diagnosis (Figure 16.19).

Endometrial hyperplasia

Endometrial hyperplasia has numerous and often confusing classification systems. The most common system in current use categorizes the hyperplasias by both architecture and presence or absence of nuclear

atypia[6]. Glandular architecture may be either simple or complex. Simple hyperplasia (Figure 16.20) consists of a minimal-to-mild increase in the gland : stroma ratio with

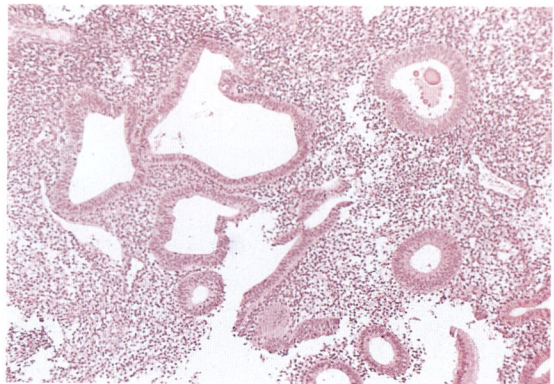

Figure 16.17 Disordered proliferation of the endometrium in anovulatory cycles may show a few cystically dilated glands mixed with a proliferative pattern. The gland : stroma ratio is not increased; the picture is not considered severe enough to be classified as hyperplasia (H & E)

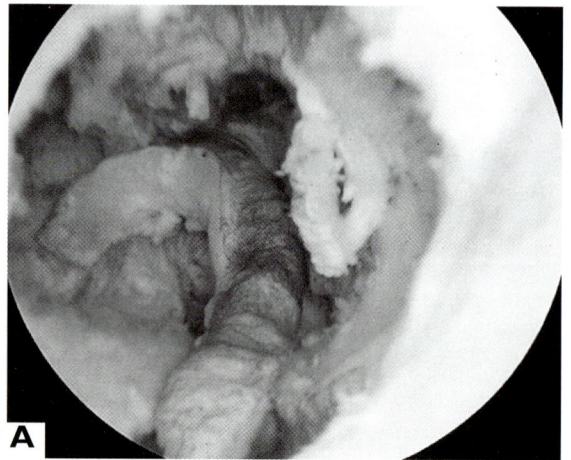

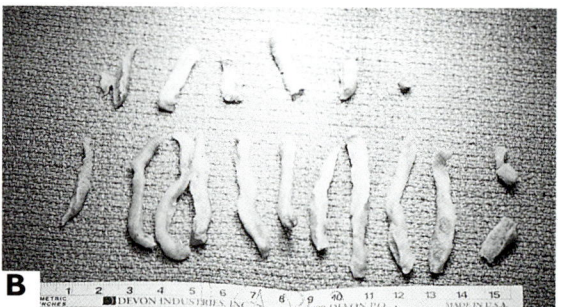

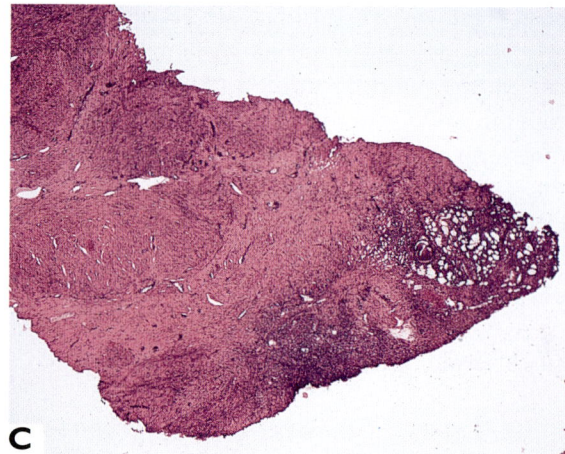

Figure 16.18 Endomyometrial resection: (**A**) view through a Storz (Culver City, CA) resectoscope, 25-F diameter with a 30° foreoblique lens, shows resection of an endomyometrial cardinal strip from the anterior uterine wall; (**B**) the resected endomyometrial strips (A and B, courtesy of Morris Wortman, MD); (**C**) low-power view of a strip removed by resection shows cautery artifact (H & E)

cystic dilatation and occasional outpouching of glands. Complex hyperplasia is used to describe more severe degrees of glandular crowding which are nevertheless insufficient to be deemed carcinoma (Figure 16.21). Atypia describes the presence of atypical glandular epithelial nuclei. Instead of the usual oval nuclei, atypical nuclei are larger and rounder, with clumping and margination of the chromatin (Figure 16.22).

There are four possible patterns of hyperplasia by this classification: simple

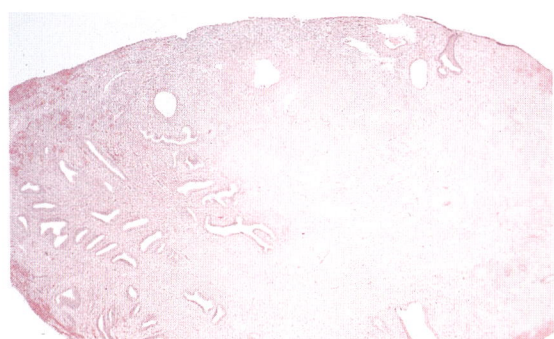

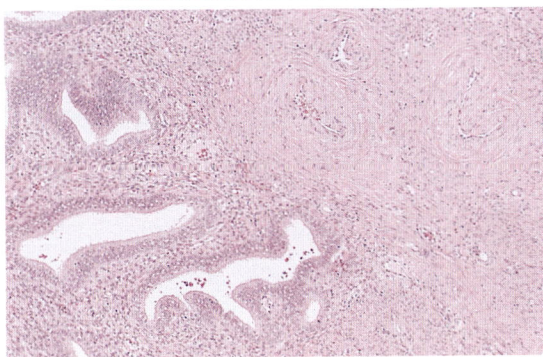

Figure 16.19 Low- (upper) and higher- (lower) power views of an endometrial polyp showing irregular stellate glands and thick vessels in the stalk (H & E)

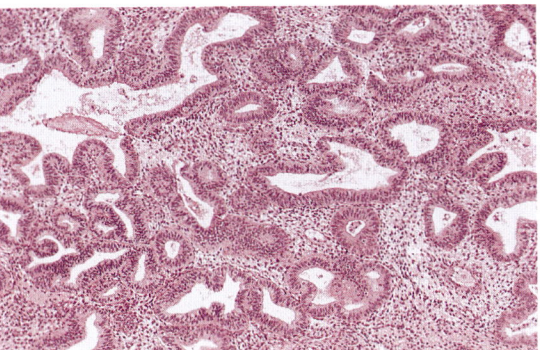

Figure 16.21 Complex hyperplasia shows increased glandular crowding (H & E)

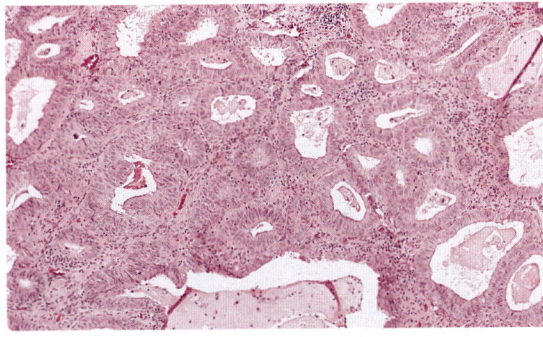

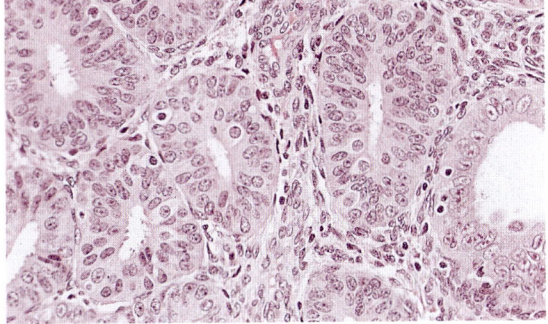

Figure 16.22 Low- (upper) and higher- (lower) power views of atypical hyperplasia (complex hyperplasia with atypia) show marked glandular crowding and nuclear atypia. The enlarged round nuclei show margination of the chromatin and prominent nucleoli (lower; H & E)

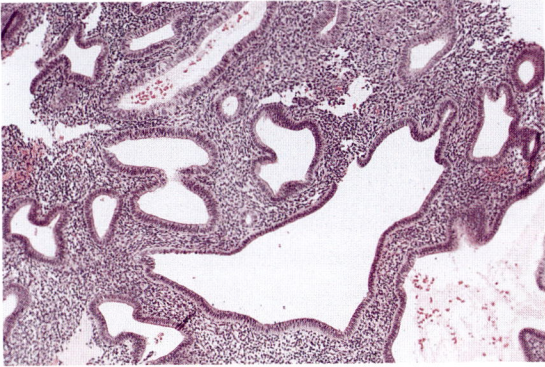

Figure 16.20 Simple hyperplasia shows mild glandular crowding (H & E)

(without atypia); simple (with atypia); complex (without atypia); and complex (with atypia). Simple hyperplasia is rarely atypical and, thus, for purposes of simplification, the terminology often consists of 'simple', 'complex' or 'atypical' hyperplasia. Atypical hyperplasia is identical to complex hyperplasia with atypia, and simple or complex hyperplasia denotes no atypia if not mentioned. The importance of this classification rests in its predictive nature. Only atypical hyperplasia has a high likelihood of being associated with either concomitant (unsampled) carcinoma or the development of carcinoma. In the study by Kurman and coworkers[6], 23% of all patients with either type of atypical hyperplasia (29% of those with complex hyperplasia with atypia) progressed to carcinoma. Knowledge of the risk of malignancy allows planning for treatment.

Endometrial carcinoma

There are several different histological subtypes of endometrial carcinoma (Table 16.2). The most prevalent is endometrioid or the usual adenocarcinoma. In the past, squamous epithelium within an endometrial adenocarcinoma led to a diagnosis of adenoacanthoma if benign in appearance, and adenosquamous carcinoma if histologically malignant. As the prognosis rests predominantly on the grade of the glandular

Table 16.2 Endometrial carcinoma: Most common histological types

Endometrioid or the usual adenocarcinoma, and variants
Endometrial adenocarcinoma with squamous differentiation
Mucinous adenocarcinoma
Clear cell adenocarcinoma
Uterine papillary serous carcinoma (UPSC)
Mixed cell type carcinoma
Undifferentiated carcinoma

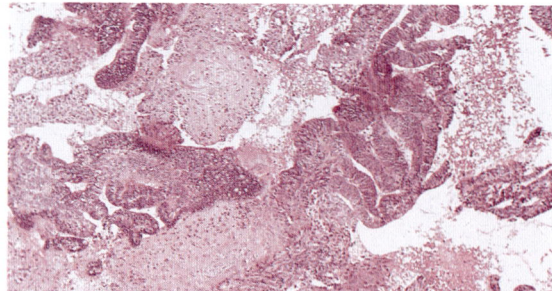
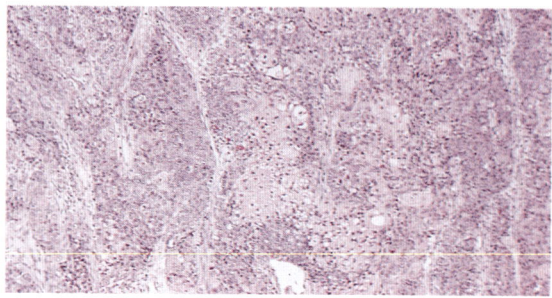

Figure 16.23 Endometrial adenocarcinoma: Well-differentiated (grade 1; upper) and poorly differentiated (grade 3; lower), with squamous differentiation (H & E)

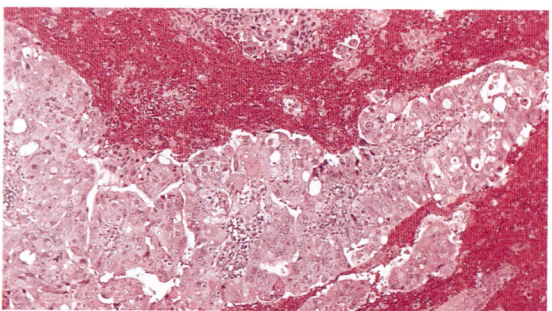

Figure 16.24 Uterine papillary serous carcinoma of the endometrium is histologically similar to ovarian papillary serous cystadenocarcinoma (H & E)

component[8], these tumors are now graded on that component with mention of squamous differentiation (Figure 16.23). For example, a diagnosis might read "Grade 2 adenocarcinoma of the endometrium with squamous differentiation". Two of the histological types – uterine papillary serous (Figure 16.24) and clear cell adenocarcinoma (Figure 16.25) – are significant for carrying a poorer prognosis than do the other types of endometrial cancer.

The current International Federation of Gynecology and Obstetrics (FIGO) staging of endometrial carcinoma is based on surgical and pathological findings (Table 16.3). For early-stage tumors, the decision whether to perform lymph node sampling at the time of hysterectomy often depends upon the tumor grade and depth of myometrial invasion. The grade used in this decision is often that assigned at initial sampling[7]. Endometrioid adenocarcinoma of the endometrium is graded in the FIGO system predominantly

according to the architecture: grade 1 is no more than 5% solid; grade 2 is 6–50% solid; and grade 3 is over 50% solid (Figures 16.26–16.28) The tumor is upgraded by one grade for signif-icant nuclear atypia. Caveats

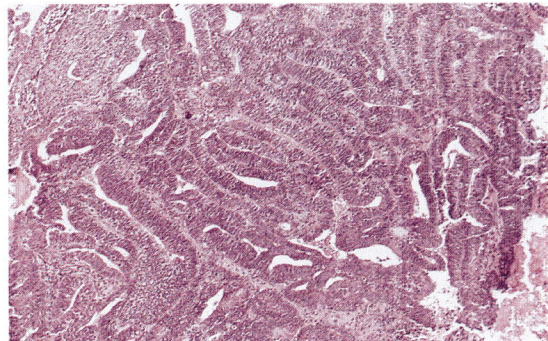

Figure 16.26 Grade 1 endometrial adenocarcinoma shows back-to-back glands without intervening stroma (H & E)

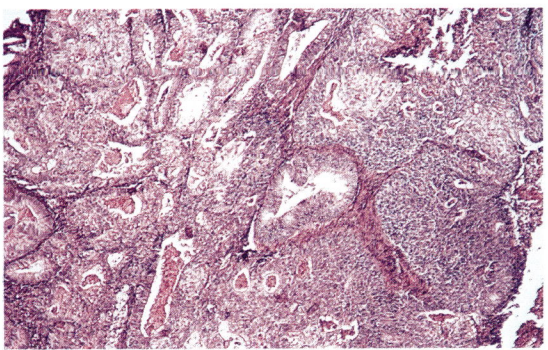

Figure 16.27 Grade 2 endometrial adenocarcinoma shows a mixture of glandular and solid areas (H & E)

Table 16.3 FIGO staging of endometrial carcinoma[9]

Stage Ia G123	Tumor limited to endometrium
Stage Ib G123	Invasion to less than one-half the myometrium
Stage Ic G123	Invasion to more than one-half the myometrium
Stage IIa G123	Endocervical glandular involvement only
Stage IIb G123	Cervical stromal invasion
Stage IIIa G123	Tumor invades serosa/adnexa and/or positive peritoneal cytology
Stage IIIb G123	Vaginal metastases
Stage IIIc G123	Metastases to pelvic and/or para-aortic lymph nodes
Stage IVa G123	Tumor invasion of bladder and/or bowel mucosa
Stage IVb	Distant metastases including intra-abdominal and/or inguinal lymph nodes

G123, grades 1, 2 or 3

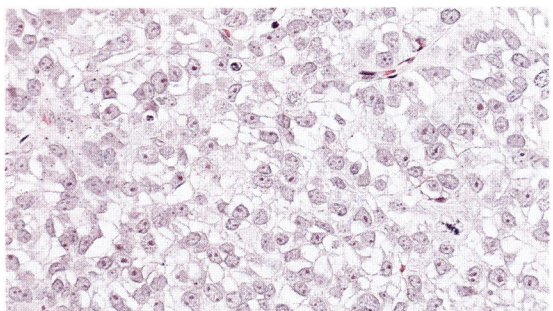

Figure 16.25 Clear cell adenocarcinoma of the endometrium (H & E)

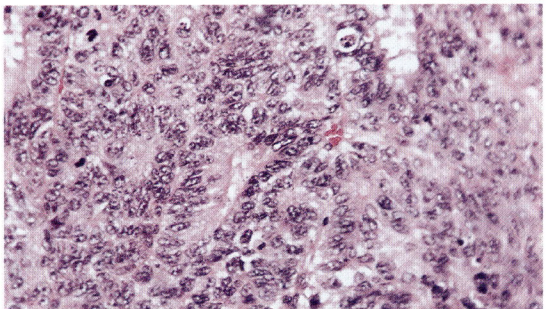

Figure 16.28 Grade 3 endometrial adenocarcinoma is predominantly solid (H & E)

include not interpreting large areas of squamous metaplasia as solid adenocarcinoma, and relying more heavily on the nuclear grade for clear cell and uterine papillary serous tumors, which have a more limited range of architecture.

Although not commonly used in staging endometrial carcinoma, hysteroscopy may assist in detecting lesions involving the cervix as well as in pinpointing the site of initial sampling.

Uterine septa / adhesions

A pathology specimen is occasionally received after hysteroscopic metroplasty or after lysis of adhesions in a patient with Asherman's syndrome. Fragments of fibromuscular tissue, often with cautery artifact, may be seen (Figure 16.29).

Myometrial lesions

Submucous leiomyoma

Submucous leiomyomas may be detected, and sometimes resected, hysteroscopically. They may be removed whole, particularly if pedunculated (Figure 16.30) but, if resected in pieces, may be difficult to distinguish from normal myometrium (Figure 16.31).

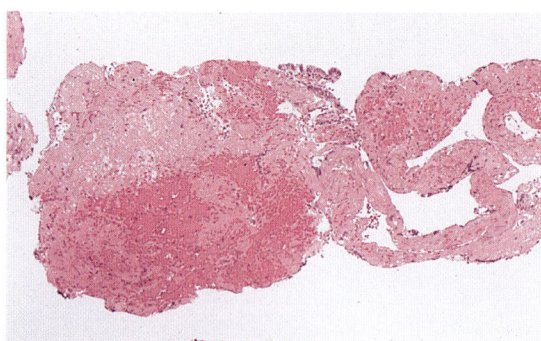

Figure 16.29 Uterine septum after hysteroscopic resection consists of fibrous tissue and endometrial fragments (H & E)

Leiomyosarcoma

Occasionally, leiomyosarcomas are detected or suspected from tissue removed hysteroscopically. The amount of tissue may be insufficient for a definitive diagnosis, which depends upon the number of mitoses per ten high-power fields as well as the presence

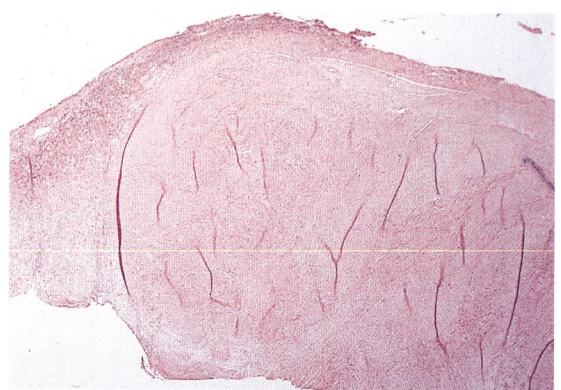

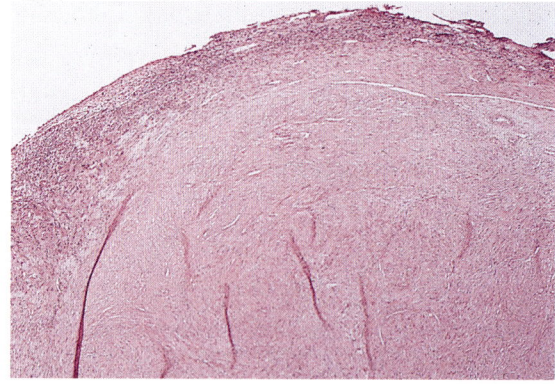

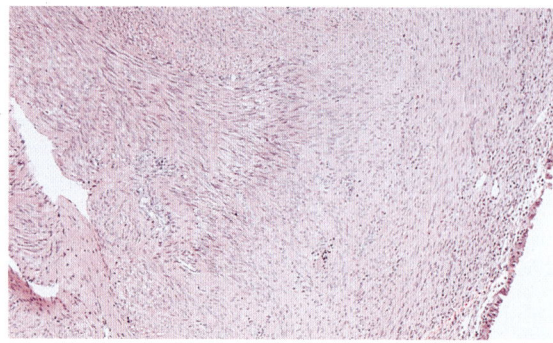

Figure 16.30 Submucous leiomyoma shows clearly the contour of the leiomyoma. Note the pressure atrophy of the endometrium (H & E)

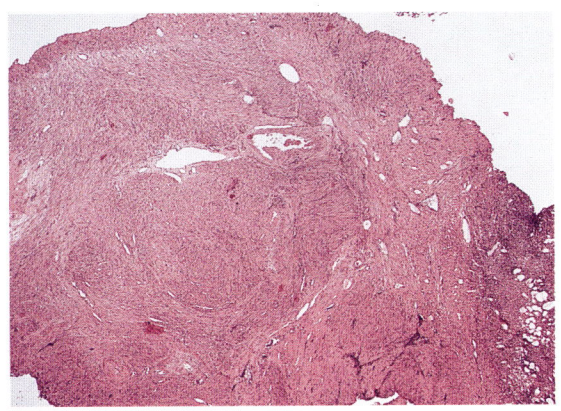

Figure 16.31 Submucous leiomyoma fragment, removed during endomyometrial resection, shows interlacing muscle bundles that are suggestive, but not diagnostic, of leiomyoma (courtesy of Morris Wortman, MD; H & E)

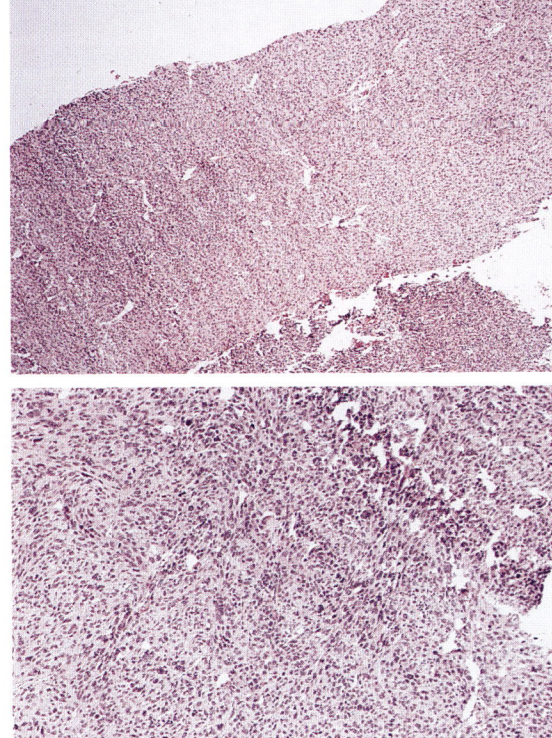

Figure 16.32 This specimen, removed during a hysteroscopic procedure, was highly suggestive of a leiomyosarcoma. This diagnosis was confirmed at hysterectomy (H & E)

or absence of atypia and necrosis (Figure 16.32).

Adenomyosis

Adenomyosis, consisting of both endometrial glands and stroma within the myometrium, can occasionally be diagnosed on a hysteroscopically obtained specimen (Figure 16.33).

Pregnancy and foreign bodies

Hysteroscopy may occasionally detect a placental polyp or retained products of conception (Figure 16.34). The most com-

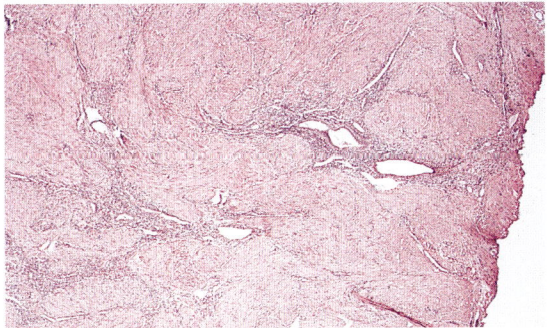

Figure 16.33 Adenomyosis consists of endometrial glands and stroma within myometrium (courtesy of Morris Wortman, MD; H & E)

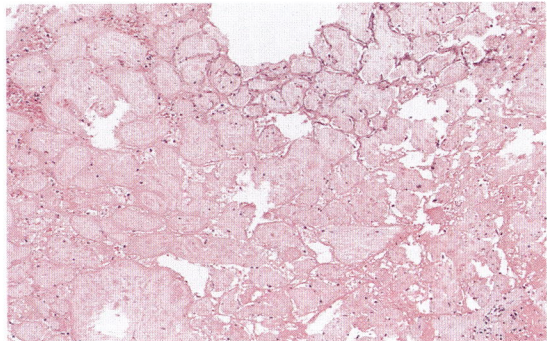

Figure 16.34 Placental polyp shows 'ghost' chorionic villi (H & E)

monly detected intrauterine foreign body is an intrauterine device (IUD), which may be difficult to remove due to retraction of the 'tail' or being imbedded in the myometrium (Figure 16.35). Removal of bone fragments[10] probably due to postintrauterine gestation and laminaria fragments[11] have been described.

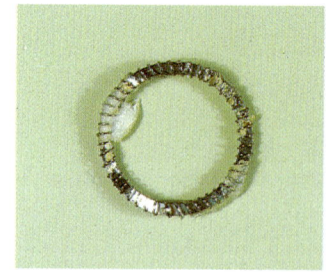

Figure 16.35 This retained IUD was imbedded in the myometrium

References

1. Noyes RW, Hertig AT, Rock J. Dating the endometrial biopsy. *Fertil Steril* 1950;1:3–25

2. Langren BM, Unden AL, Diczfalusy E. Hormonal profile of the cycle in 68 normally menstruating women. *Acta Endocrinol Copenh* 1980;94:89–98

3. Nuovo MA, Nuovo GJ, McCaffrey R, *et al.* Endometrial polyps in postmenopausal patients receiving tamoxifen. *Int J Gynecol Pathol* 1989;8:125–31

4. Heller D. *The Endometrium: A Clinico-pathologic Approach.* New York: Igaku-Shoin Medical Publishers, 1994:76–80

5. Wortman M, Daggett A. Hysteroscopic endomyometrial resection: A new technique for the treatment of menorrhagia. *Obstet Gynecol* 1994;83:295–8

6. Kurman RJ, Kaminsky PF, Norris HJ. The behavior of endometrial hyperplasia: A long-term study of "untreated" hyperplasia in 170 patients. *Cancer* 1985;56:403–12

7. Heller D, Drosinos S, Westhoff C. Accuracy of tumor grade assigned at initial endometrial sampling (Letter). *Int J Gynecol Obstet* 1994;47:301–2

8. Zaino RJ, Kurman RJ. Squamous differentiation in carcinoma of the endometrium: A critical appraisal of adenoacanthoma and adenosquamous carcinoma. *Semin Diagn Pathol* 1988;5:154–71

9. Creasman WT. New gynecologic cancer staging. *Obstet Gynecol* 1990;75:287–8

10. Marcus SF, Bhattacharya J, Williams G, *et al.* Endometrial ossification: A cause of secondary infertility. *Am J Obstet Gynecol* 1994;170:1381–3

11. Borgatta L, Barad D. Prolonged retention of laminaria fragments: An unusual complication of laminaria usage. *Obstet Gynecol* 1991;78: 988–90

Epilogue

Hysteroscopy has achieved its proper place in modern gynecology. The early problems associated with its performance have been solved with new instrumentation and the safe use of CO_2 gas and / or low-viscosity fluids to distend the uterine cavity with simple and effective methods of delivery. Light sources have been improved and miniature cameras with excellent resolution introduced, adding to the armamentarium and safety of the technique. Video hysteroscopy is now a routine method of evaluation and treatment. Office hysteroscopy has been made possible with simpler instrumentation and endoscopes that do not require cervical dilatation, thereby reducing patient inconvenience and discomfort, saving physician time and inconvenience, and eliminating the bureaucracy entailed with the use of ambulatory surgical centers or operating suites. The diagnostic applications of hysteroscopy are well-defined, enabling evaluation not only of structural abnormalities such as myomas, polyps, anatomical anomalies and pathological scars that distort the uterine cavity, but also the different changes that the endometrium may undergo, whether benign, premalignant and / or malignant.

The therapeutic applications of hysteroscopy have expanded and are also well-defined. The uterine septum can be treated transcervically, thereby supplanting abdominal metroplasty; submucous leiomyomas can be safely resected without the need for a laparotomy; and intrauterine adhesions can be divided with greater precision to provide an improved reproductive outcome compared with the previous blind or more invasive methods of treatment. Tubal cannulation for cornual occlusion is now the first step in the evaluation and treatment, allowing the selection of only those patients with fibrotic occlusions that will benefit most from microsurgical resection and anastomosis. Endometrial ablation is a viable alternative to hysterectomy for women with dysfunctional uterine bleeding that is unresponsive to hormonal treatment.

Finally, new and promising hysteroscopic applications are on the horizon. Technological improvements and adaptation of various techniques may eventually prove beneficial for the use of hysteroscopy and include embryoscopy, direct visual delivery of gametes, zygotes or embryos into the uterine cavity, and a practical method of observing and evaluating the intratubal epithelium from the uterine side.

Hysteroscopy has a well-earned place in gynecology today and should be used in patients who may benefit from intrauterine visualization.

Index